The Dementia Diet

Slowing Neurocognitive Decline
Or
How Not To Lose Your Memories

Dr. Christopher Maloney, N.D.

ISBN: 9781798867327

DEDICATION

To the gut wrenching moment when I forgot something really important.
Despite the terror, it was a wake-up call for me to help others. My work is
for all of us who suffer together.

CONTENTS

ACKNOWLEDGMENTS

I want to thank our medical and community support teams. In an increasingly harried and complicated world they do a wonderful job. While I will critique their work I am truly thankful. I would also like to thank my family, my friends and patients for being there with love, support and fruit salads. There are not words enough to thank my wife.

Preface

When I was fifteen, I found out I would get Alzheimer's disease and die without a memory. Not in a doctor's office, in my science class. No, it wasn't because of a family history. It was because of my fingerprints.

That's right. My fingerprints said I would die with no memory. In a groundbreaking study, A New York neurologist had found that people with certain fingerprints had a very high chance of getting Alzheimer's disease. The deadly fingerprints included a lot of loops. Mine were the worst in the class. I remember looking at my fingers and thinking I was doomed.

What I got that sunny day in science class, surrounded by my fellow pimply teens with their still immature brains was a terrible fear of Alzheimer's disease, mnemophobia (nemm-o-phobia) a terror of memory loss. It's a terror that afflicts many people, especially as we get older. A twenty-year-old might joke about not being able to remember what they did on Friday night, but once you cross into your late forties, it's no laughing matter.

Mnemophobia can also be the fear of bad memories, the ones we'd rather forget. We all want to keep our good memories, but there's always that awkward, room silencing fart or hurtful comment we'd all like to erase. I suppose most of us wouldn't mind selective Alzheimer's disease, as long as we could pick what was lost. So we're both fearful of losing our precious memories and fearful someone will remember our embarrassing moments from years ago. We humans have a complex relationship with our memories.

All these years I've held onto my adolescent fear of memory loss, a painful knowledge like a crystalline splinter waiting to torment me if I forget my car keys or the name of a celebrity. It troubles me at the moment it happens, like a shadow crossing the window of my soul, but I conveniently forget to follow up later. Why confirm the inevitable? If I ignore it perhaps I can somehow avoid the fate written on my own palm.

Only after reading an amazing essay by a professor who is losing her memory did I finally sit down. I needed to make myself face my fear and see if I could do something about it.

The professor's essay didn't convince me because of its brilliance. What convinced me was that it took the professor nine months to write those few pages. I realized by the time I started really losing my own memory it might be too late to do the research I needed. By the time I needed to write this book for myself and all of you, I'll be too far gone to write it.

If you're a new reader, you should know I'm on a mission. Since my colon cancer diagnosis in 2015, I've written books to help humanity. So writing this book on memory for me is an exercise in optimism that I'll live long enough to need it. It's also an offering to all of you who may have the good fortune to live long enough to suffer through memory loss.

More importantly, I want all of us to not lose our memories now. We must actively resist the loss of our amazing mind playgrounds, our mental home movies, and our internal surround-sound photo albums. When people run from a burning home, the only things they pick up are their memories. Memories are more precious to us than money and second only to our loved ones. We should know how to keep our memories safe in our heads.

So that's what I want to explain in this short book: how to keep your memories.

I'm going to talk about what memory is, how the brain functions to keep memories. Then I'm going to go through how we lose our memories. We'll look at how to make your memory stronger. Finally I'll give you what I'm doing personally to keep from losing my mind one memory at a time.

When I started looking at memory research, I started to get more and more confused. Nothing seemed to agree. There were world authorities contradicting other world authorities. I couldn't tell what was true. Maybe researching dementia too much starts to make you feel like you're getting dementia. But then I realized I'd stumbled across a silent power struggle between how we treat and even how we define memory loss. In the last ten years experts have been trying to rewrite everything we think we know about the brain and memory. So I'll do my best to guide you through a massive earthquake in how we think about memory loss.

Please don't take my word for anything. Every month there are 30,000 medical articles published, and no one has read them all. I'm going to make clear that your mind is unique, so no expert can say for certain what you need. When you read this book, take the information to someone you trust to help you make medical decisions. Then make your own choices. Please don't assume my personal plan is perfect for you, as if what I'm doing would work as well for an alcoholic in Omaha or an octogenarian tea drinker in England. It doesn't. I don't even know if it will work for me. But I'm choosing to roll the dice with the best information I have, increasing my odds of keeping my mind (I hope.)

In the end, none of us knows when we will die. I hope this book gives some of you the tools to live longer, healthier, more memory rich lives.

1 What Do We Know About Memory Loss?

If you think you're losing your memories, you're not alone. A lot of people are losing their memories worldwide. Right now 50 million people live with dementia or Alzheimer's disease. By 2030, the number will be 75 million.[i] If the experts are right, by 2050 more than 132 million people have Alzheimer's disease or dementia.[ii]

But these numbers fluctuate depending on who you read. The new estimates are 30% higher than they were a few years ago. The experts are basing their estimates on how much dementia is being diagnosed in central Asia or places where there isn't a good medical system. So we are just guesstimating. Even the information we have within the United States varies widely from state to state. And the definitions of how we determine what is dementia and what is Alzheimer's disease may be changing.

ALZHEIMER'S DISEASE VS. DEMENTIA

We have two different diseases, dementia and Alzheimer's disease, that both mean you're losing your mind one memory at a time.

What's the difference?

Historically, it was that dementia was more general and Alzheimer's disease was more specific. Think of it as if dementia represented all sandwiches in the world and Alzheimer's disease was just peanut butter and jelly. A peanut butter sandwich is a type of sandwich, but you could also have a ham and cheese. So Alzheimer's was just one type of dementia, the most common type. There were other, more exotic kinds of dementias that you could also get.

All that changed recently. The word dementia has bad associations. We wouldn't want patients to feel badly about losing their minds. So dementia has been replaced in the new medical textbooks by newer, less derogatory terms (I voted for memory-challenged, but they went with mild and major neurocognitive disorder).

While I understand the memory doctors want to make people feel better about the diagnosis, I'm going to keep using the term dementia in this book. The simple reason is that we don't have studies yet on "minor or major neurocognitive disorder." Those terms just got made up by well-meaning experts.

The medical information that we have is about dementia. So rather than throwing up our hands and waiting another decade for new research, I think we need to move forward with dementia until they come out with new studies based on the new terms.

WHAT IS ALZHEIMER'S DISEASE NOW?

The other term we use all the time, Alzheimer's disease (AD), used to mean something very specific.

In 1906 Alois Alzheimer gave a lecture on memory loss and showed other doctors the specific brain changes that he thought caused that memory loss. These were the plaques and tangles that most of us vaguely know about as the telltale signs of brain issues. That was Alzheimer's disease.

Now the very definition of Alzheimer's disease is being changed and experts are arguing about what it should be.

Spoiler alert: it turns out Alzheimer might have been wrong about those brain changes causing memory loss.

Alzheimer's disease (AD) has always been a diagnosis made

after every other kind of dementia has been ruled out. But the differences between AD and diseases like vascular (blood vessel caused) dementia are becoming less clear over time. One review showed that 90% of Alzheimer's patients also have blood vessel problems.[iii] So if you've got both, does having AD really make a difference?

Spoiler alert: we don't know.

The goal of separating out Alzheimer's disease from the other dementias was to find different, better treatments for people who weren't having strokes in their heads. But after decades, we know the majority of dementia patients (insert the proper politically correct current term here if you'd like) have symptoms that include both Alzheimer's disease and other dementias. In other words, almost all dementia patients are "mixed dementia patients" with multiple disease processes at the same time. At least they have "mixed dementia" now. The experts will likely change that derogatory term to "funky major cognitive disorder" or whatever else they're planning to use in the future to make sure no one feels bad.

While I make fun of the name changes, we do need to dramatically change how we think about memory loss. Rather than helping us solve the problem, our old definitions are slowing our ability to treat dementia patients effectively today.[iv]

I think we need to go farther than just changing the term dementia. It's time to recognize that the way we think about Alzheimer's disease and dementia, diagnose it, and are trying to treat it, doesn't help us. We need to let go of those names along with changing entirely our way of thinking about memory loss.

Going forward, I'm going to talk mostly about dementia, but please include "and Alzheimer's disease" if I don't put it in. The overlap is too great to separate them at this point. I'm also going to discuss how we diagnose memory loss and Alzheimer's disease because - while I don't like the term – Alzheimer's disease is the scariest and most misunderstood form of dementia.

2 What Do We Know About The Brain?

Despite lots of literature about how the brain functions, we know a surprisingly small amount about the brain and memory loss.

The problem is that researchers can't go poking about in a person's brain, taking pieces out and putting them back. Medical ethics prevents us from monkeying around in the human brain. You can't do a brainectomy and then ask patients how they feel.

Yes, we do bad things with the brains of other animals, but this doesn't give us great information on human memory loss. No one can ask a mouse if missing a part of its brain makes everything smell like lemons or if removing a little sliver took its memory of its best friend from mouse middle school.

CATS, MRIS, AND MONEYS

But what about all those big, expensive brain scans? You know, your CATS, MRIs, your MONEYs? They look impressive, but they aren't that specific. There's a reason that experts talk about "regions of the brain" rather than "brain fold four, upper right hand pinkie finger tightener." Our information is pretty general.

The best way we have to check on the brain's activity is through a functional MRI, which gives us a picture of which areas of the brain are the most active. The MRI tells us which areas are consuming the most oxygen. We've also got a very general map of an average person's brain (not sure who). So we have a sense of which area likely does what, but we really don't have a map of your specific brain. It's like using a map from the 1940's to try and navigate the city of Cleveland today. Sometimes you'll be right, but chances are you're going to miss an overpass or two.

We also don't have a good sense of how the average brain functions over time. The two kinds of measures we take are very short term (seconds) and very long term (after months or years). So again, we're trying to figure out how memory functions based on snapshots. It would be like trying to get to know your new grandchild or nephew based on a few photos. Sure, you can get a sense of things, but you really don't have a full picture of what goes on and why that child does or doesn't remember you.[v]

In the average brain different parts of the brain light up when we do different things. Mapping those lit-up areas can tell us a lot about average human's behavior. The key word is average. That scan may not apply at all to you or me.

BUT AREN'T WE ALL ALIKE? NOT AT ALL

Trained individuals may have entirely different brain responses than untrained individuals. For example, hook me and a NASCAR driver up to brain scan helmets and put us in a convertible heading for a cliff at 200 miles an hour (in kilometers that's...wicked fast). A trained NASCAR driver's brain would react to traveling in a car at 200 mph by lighting up her trained motor pathways to her arms and legs, preparing to control the car. My brain's response to traveling in a convertible at 200 mph toward a cliff might be to light up the pathways for screaming at the top of my lungs and possibly releasing my bladder, resulting in me wetting myself.

But put us in a medical situation and the scans reverse. The same NASCAR driver's brain might light up with confusion when she's asked about the deltoid ligament. For me that question would set off in my brain a cascade of associated patients, memories of med school exams, and ultimately a visual memory of where it sits in the body and how to check it to see if it's been torn. Completely different results for the same situation.

Over our lifetimes we train our brains, and part of that training determines which memories are connected to other memories. Each of our brains contain unique memories and unique memory maps, so we can never know for certain how something is stored until we lose it.

In the scans, the lit up brain areas tell us which areas are getting more oxygen. More oxygen usually means more activity, but not necessarily. Different brains need different amounts of oxygen, and brains deprived of oxygen over time can learn to function on less. Brain scans of high-altitude Himalayan Sherpas show much less oxygen use than someone living at sea level. An elderly person with chronic lung issues might show similar changes, giving a false impression of less brain function. Granpa may still have his memories of the fifties, he may just be better at conserving his oxygen so they don't show up on his MRI.

The map of the average brain is based on where things are likely to be in the brain. But just as a road map may not tell you about a road closure or a new shortcut, the brain map doesn't tell us why one person can still recall most of her life while another person can't even remember what a toaster does. They may both be missing the same part of the brain, but one of the two has managed to work around it. So when doctors discuss brain scans, they can make it sound like what they are saying is established when much of brain science is still exploration.

DOES BRAIN LOSS DETERMINE MEMORY LOSS?

Memory loss gives us a picture of the brain in crisis, but we don't know how it functions when the brain is at peak capacity. Currently our best guess is that the anatomy of the brain, all the bits we can see, affects how we remember. But it doesn't determine how well we remember. The anatomy of our brains, and the loss of that anatomy (tangles, holes, or plaques) does not determine how much memory we lose. Having big holes makes a difference, but there are seniors out there who have brains that look like swiss cheese and who are still functioning normally. They terrify their doctors with horrifying MRIs, but then go off and live a normal life.

How is this possible? Our brains function on a level that is much more complex than any computer. A computer has many, many, on/off switches. But the human brain has many, many on/kind of on/somewhat off switches. Imagine a computer as a vast room full of regular light bulbs, all flickering on and off. Now imagine the human brain as the same vast room but with all the light bulbs on dimmer switches. Some of them are all the way on, some are all the way off. But the majority are somewhere in between. So instead of a very high number of on/off light bulbs in our brains, we have an almost infinite number of dimmers at various levels of dimness. That's how complicated the human brain is compared to a super computer. And that's why we don't really understand how some people can function normally with what looks like devastating damage in their brain while others with nearly normal brains are seriously compromised.

3 Does It Run In Your Family?

"Does it run in your family?"

You know the drill. If you're family has dementia in it, then you're more likely to get dementia. It's like Uncle Charlie's bum ticker. If you inherited it, all you can do is shrug your shoulders.

THE ALL GENETICS CROWD

A few researchers still hold the view that dementia is almost entirely genetic. They base this on population-based studies, on the fact that close relatives have higher risk of getting dementia, and using the studies on identical twins that put the genetic risk of dementia higher than 60%. Of all the genetic risk factors, these researchers estimate that just the APOE genetic variation accounts for more than half of the dementia cases.[vi]

We could ignore this minority of researchers except that one of the authors of this point of view is Dr. Wesson Ashford, who heads the screening board of the Alzheimer's Foundation and is the senior editor of the Journal of Alzheimer's Disease. His assumption that APOE is causative for dementia has yet to be proven, and the treatments based on APOE as a cause for dementia have been shown to be useless.[vii] If you look at all the new genetic markers including APOE, the Mayo Clinic is clear that "these genes are risk factors, not direct causes."[viii] Even Dr. Ashford recently wrote about "encouraging positive health behaviors"[ix] to avoid dementia. Not something you would expect from an "it's all genetics" guy.

THE MIXED CROWD

Unlike many diseases, the majority of memory researchers agree that Alzheimer's disease (dementia is too broad a term for genetics) is almost entirely not genetic. But for a select few, their genes do increase their risk.

The unlucky few have one of a small number of genes that increase their risk of Alzheimer's disease. These include APP, PS-1, PS-2, and APOE4. I'm sure there are more, and those of you who have one of these genes have our sympathy.

So sorry you've got the genes of doom.

Except that having one of these genes does not mean you will get Alzheimer's disease. It just increases your risk.

Take the most common of the genes, APOE4. The Dominantly Inherited Alzheimer Network (DIAN) monitors patients with this gene. They found that young people with the gene had more amyloid plaque formation earlier in their lives.[x]

Which is bad, but doesn't necessarily mean they will develop early dementia. Amyloid plaques don't directly correspond with memory loss.

TRYING TO KEEP GENETICS RELEVANT

Rather than finding more conclusive genetic links, researchers are now combining genetics with biomarkers and brain scans. They conclude "that ApoE4 could be at least partially responsible for some of the observed disease heterogeneity."[xi] So having the genes could possibly affect the disease? That's not a very strong statement from people who used to think genes caused dementia.

The problem with the genetic model for dementia is that it didn't hold up in real life. If people had ApoE4 and poor memory, they performed more poorly on tests than regular patients. But those with ApoE4 and normal memory performed better on tests than regular patients. The normal-memory ApoE4 patients also had a larger than usual hippocampus, the part of the brain most affected by Alzheimer's disease.[xii] So the brains of some ApoE4 patients seems to have compensated for the ApoE4 gene.

While it may now be confusing what to expect if you have ApoE4, that confusion is actually extremely hopeful. If you go to the DIAN website, they have this message for just-diagnosed genetic patients. "There is currently no treatment that can prevent or delay the progression of AD, and no new treatments have been approved in over ten years."[xiii] All the current treatments for dementia are so bad France won't even pay for them. So basically the reason to sign up for DIAN is to allow your own deterioration to be monitored for the possible benefit of future generations.

But the number of people with DIAN proven, genetically-linked dementia is low. "The disease affects less than 1% of the total population of people with Alzheimer's."[xiv] So it's nice to know that 99% of dementia and Alzheimer's disease isn't genetic. Even for those who do have the genes, having them just acts as an increased risk factor rather than a life sentence.

For me, not having a genetic smoking gun for Alzheimer's gives me some peace of mind. I still haven't gotten over the fear that my fingerprints might not get me. But the reality that almost all dementia is not genetic says that there is something I can do in my lifetime to avoid losing my mind.

If you've been diagnosed with memory loss and told it might be genetic, please realize you haven't doomed your relatives to your fate because of your genetics. So take a moment to let go of that particular guilt. And yes, they should still get tested, monitored, and be careful with their lifestyles.

4 Do You Have Memory Loss?

YES.

If you think you have memory loss, you do. But should you be worried it's progressive? If you think it's progressive, it's progressive. Get checked.

Why? Because almost all the time it's not dementia. Only 18% of cases are early dementia.

As you get older depression can also be a sign of dementia, so don't assume you're just depressed. It can be hard to tell what's what even with a medical degree. Even doctors have to rely on "rules of thumb" to decide whether to send someone on to a specialist.[xv]

BUT...

If you think you're losing your memory, chances are that your memory isn't that bad yet. You still have good metamemory, an awareness that your memory isn't as good as it once was.[xvi] This awareness differs between individuals and no doctor can truly assess if you really have decreased memory as long as your memory still meets certain basic functional standards.

Think of it like going in and saying that you don't walk as well as you used to. Your doctor watches you walk and says you look fine. After badgering her, you get a referral to a walking specialist. The specialist hooks you up to a walking machine and again says everything looks good. But you know you don't walk as well as you used to, because you did years of gymnastics on a balance beam and now you have to separate your legs wider than your hips to feel stable. You feel less stable, but because your personal standard of function is so much higher than the basic standard of function, you look fine on all the standardized walking tests.

The same problem applies to memory. If once upon a time you remembered every family member, every in-law, and all your grandchildren's favorite things, forgetting which grandchild likes Pooh bear and which prefers Paddington bear can be very troubling. But it's not going to show up on any memory test as a deficiency to be worried about. Not until you can't recall your in-laws or even your children's names will you be considered non-functional. It's a very low bar, and the result is a huge gap between what patients experience as memory loss and doctors define as memory loss.

FUNCTIONAL MEMORY LOSS VS. SUBJECTIVE COGNITIVE DECLINE

The gap between losing your memory and meeting the diagnosis of memory loss means that you can be diagnosed with functional memory loss. This diagnosis unfortunately allows clinicians to ignore progressive memory loss. Functional memory loss is simply your subjective over-focus on "normal aging" memory loss. Normal aging models predict that dementia will double every five years after sixty. That same model found that dementia rates jumped to 70% between 90 and 95. But people who make it to 100 in Sweden only have a 40% dementia rate. So I guess they haven't read the "normal aging" studies.[xvii]

Since in functional memory loss you likely don't show dramatic memory loss, the specialists will treat you for anxiety around memory loss or recommend psychological coping strategies rather than consider you for trials or other interventions. Functional memory loss means you worry too much about your memory, which is fine.

If you are older than seventy, then instead of functional memory loss you may get diagnosed with subjective cognitive decline. If this sounds almost exactly like functional memory loss, that would be correct. It's subjective, meaning in your opinion your memory is worse, but there are no objective signs of memory loss. Since you're older, the doctors recognize that memory loss can be a part of being older. So you get a different diagnosis. But the results are the same. You don't have anything they need to be concerned about treating.

IS MEMORY TESTING OBJECTIVE OR SUBJECTIVE?

Memory loss, even with the most commonly used and tested screening, (the Mini-Mental State Examination or MMSE) can be subjective. The MMSE tests for today's date, something even healthy adults are often confused about. Almost all the MMSE questions are verbal. A person would lose only two points and be declared mentally fit even if she were completely unable to use her physical body to accomplish any task.

It brings to mind the story of "a retired philosophy professor...who can no longer bathe, dress, or feed himself, but directs canonical philosophy discussions with visiting former colleagues."[xviii] How well would he score on the MMSE?

The questions asked are also skewed to long term brain pathways. Again a person could pass with virtually no short term memory.[xix] Improvements on the MMSE, which were available online for free, were pulled off the internet after the MMSE authors sued for copyright infringement.[xx] As a result, other researchers are creating tests that won't have the same scale or questions as the MMSE. While this satisfies the greed of the MMSE authors, it means that future studies won't be comparable to those done up until now. Greed is costing decades of beneficial research results. So keep in mind how varied and subjective memory testing is as we go forward.

Can we prove that memory testing is completely subjective? Almost. When Medicare tracks Alzheimer diagnoses across the United States, the reported rate of Alzheimer's varies. It doesn't just vary by a few percentage points, which you might expect (older population or less active). It varies by almost half. If you live in Arizona, you're chances of getting diagnosed with Alzheimer's disease is over 40% less than if you live in Texas.[xxi] Before you move to Arizona, all that means is that the rate of diagnosis varies wildly. The screening tests are that subjective.

MCI: REAL MEMORY LOSS

Only if you are diagnosed with mild cognitive impairment (MCI) do you have recognized memory loss that doctors can measure. MCI is the beginning stages of dementia or Alzheimer's disease. This diagnosis should be limited to those few people who could benefit from experimental treatments since we currently have nothing proven that treats or slows the process. But since patients who know about memory loss also know that functional or subjective loss isn't a "real" diagnosis, they may pressure their doctors to diagnose them with MCI even though they really don't have measurable memory loss. In turn, this skews any studies we have on memory loss drugs, because some of those "benefiting" may not have had any real measurable loss when they started the trials.

MCI memory loss usually includes a brain scan showing changes that could indicate early Alzheimer's disease. For many doctors, MCI is the same as early Alzheimer's, while other doctors use the term more loosely to include any measurable memory loss.

CONFIRMING WITH A BRAIN SCAN?

Is the scan conclusive evidence of MCI? No. The difficulty is that brain scans of normal older brains without memory loss can also show all the signs of early Alzheimer's disease.

In other words, you could have functional or subjective memory loss combined with a brain scan that shows brain changes. These results could indicate MCI but the brain changes may also have been there for years with no memory issues.

So you could be diagnosed with early Alzheimer's disease without really having early Alzheimer's disease. The rates of misdiagnosis are very high, with about a quarter of normal older patients showing scan changes similar to early Alzheimer's and another 20% showing possible stroke damage. But none of those individuals experienced memory loss when questioned or tested. In some cases normal older adults can have brain scans that show what we assume would be extremely advanced Alzheimer's changes without any loss in memory function.

The best news is for people with subjective cognitive decline. Your rates of progressing to early Alzheimer's disease are about the same as the rest of the older population. As long as the memory loss isn't particularly concerning to your doctor, the brain can compensate for some memory loss by engaging other pathways.

IS YOUR DOCTOR CONCERNED?

If your memory loss is concerning to your doctor, then that concern is as accurate as any test. If it's particularly concerning, then it's actually the most accurate measure of whether you are at risk for worsening memory.[xxii] Which should be obvious, but all this testing can get confusing. **The best measure of how bad your memory loss is comes from having a trained person talk to you and assess just how bad it has become.**

TRYING TO GET MORE HELP

For younger people diagnosed with functional memory loss (FML) the long term outcomes are usually a stable memory, which should be good news. But that doesn't mean your memory improves, leading to lots of frustration with doctors. Most FML sufferers cycle through medical offices and remain stable for decades without improvement. The most common sign of FML is greatly increased stress, so get ready to hear that a great deal about lowering your stress levels. FML can strike early, with up to 29% of patients as young as 24 complaining of some level of memory loss.[xxiii] That's decades of concern without any resolution if you pursue standard medical channels. Hopefully this book will give you some more useful places to focus your energy.

BUT SHOULDN'T YOU GET TESTING ANYWAY?

Not necessarily.

While we argue about definitions and testing, the reality is that no one is doing the follow-up work on whether early testing for memory loss results in better outcomes. We have early testing for things like heart disease or cancer screening, and generally those outcomes are better if you screen people earlier. But when you look at memory testing, early screening doesn't really show up. A 2013 review found that we don't even have a consistent screening tool used by most doctors (The MMSE is the most frequent, but it's not a standard.) The ones we do have are better at detecting outright dementia much better than mild decline. There are no studies that follow-up memory screening for any important outcomes like disease progression, hospitalization, or future diagnoses. We literally have no information on whether being screened early or often for memory loss will be helpful to you at all.[xxiv]

5 Can We Do More Harm Than Good?

Even though the science about the brain and memory is debatable. It can be both terrifying and sound very final.

Let's look at the proof when I was fifteen years old that I was going to get Alzheimer's disease.

My science teacher terrified me with this fact, looking at my hand and commented on how it applied to me personally. Then she went on lecturing about the brain as if she had somehow not just given me a death sentence.

A NOCEBO EFFECT

In our adolescent years, we tend to fixate on things like predestined doom. In the back of my mind, the fingerprint destiny has always been there, like a dull toothache. If I forgot something, I might look at my fingers, as if my fingerprints themselves were mutating, getting worse. Talk about a casual curse, or a "nocebo effect" in medical terms. The opposite of placebo, nocebo is when doctors mistakenly tell you that you're worse off than you are. The result can be extremely stressful, and even life threatening.

Only when I decided to write this book did I have the courage to go back and look to see if there really was a study on fingerprints. All this time I might have been the victim of my science teacher having read a tabloid article in the grocery store checkout line.

While there is no official phobia of reading about your own imminent death in a grocery store checkout line, a fear of bad news would be diurno-phobia (common enough these days). So all these years I could have been living in fear of some hack journalist's need to sell tabloid newspapers, too scared to look up the truth.

Was it just a tabloid story?

No. I wasn't so lucky.

That fingerprint study really does exist (cue sinking heart, bitten fingernails, curse family and genetics). A simple medline search of "fingerprints, Alzheimer's" finds the original study.

THE FINGERPRINT OF DOOM

My doom was sealed by Dr. Weinreb in 1986.

Dr. H. J. Weinreb was a New York neurologist who rocked the neurology world with his simple solution for diagnosing dementia very early in life. Weinreb said his fingerprint analysis could find dementia and Alzheimer's disease with "84% sensitivity and 63% specificity."[xxv] That means it can spot most future dementia and that more than half the time that dementia will be Alzheimer's disease. Those are good numbers. Heck, those are great numbers. Weinreb's fingerprint test outperforms our current modern MRI tests.

Was it a fluke test? A mistake?

Nope.

Not only did Dr. Weinreb do the original study, he repeated his study with a larger group to show his results could be replicated. His second study made international medical news, and I got to hear the bad news myself in science class between dissecting frog legs and coloring in arm.

SO AM I DOOMED? NOT QUITE.

As you might expect, I wasn't the only person troubled by a palm of doom. As they tried to figure out their fates, other researchers found they couldn't repeat Weinreb's palm reading. Follow-up studies failed to confirm Dr. Weinreb's suspicion about fingerprints. But those negative studies never reached my science classroom. It's a case of positive research bias, where the crazy first study gets lots of publicity but nobody cares if it's proven not true in later studies.

The problem with Weinreb's studies was that they weren't double-blind, only single-blind. A single-blind study is when patients don't know what they're getting, a double-blind study is when both the doctors and the patients don't know what's going on. Dr. Weinreb knew what he was looking for in the fingerprints of his patients, and he found it. But other doctors who were blinded about who had dementia didn't find fingerprints helpful in figuring it out. In multiple studies, researchers didn't find a significant difference in fingerprints between people with dementia and people who didn't have dementia. So if the doctors didn't know who had Alzheimer's disease, the fingerprints didn't predict anything.[xxvi]

It's a case of Dr. Weinreb seeing a pattern in the fingerprints of his patients because he wanted to see a pattern there. His results are relevant to today's memory loss research because many researchers today discuss finding brain "fingerprints" predicting dementia in the MRIs of their patients.

6 Will We Find The Fingerprint of Doom?

So Dr. Weinreb was wrong, my fingerprints won't take my memories. I followed up on his life, because I wanted to know more about this man who haunted me for decades. He graduated from Reed College, ten blocks from where I lived as a child. Just before his death, Dr. Weinreb forgot to fill out his own life insurance paperwork, leaving his wife destitute (the court case is public online). So I suspect he was personally motivated to figure out a fast way to predict memory issues. I wonder if he had a lot of loops on his own hands. I can feel bad that he probably suffered from the thing he'd spent his life researching. But I can still feel a little resentful that Dr. Weinreb terrified me for years.

SO WILL WE FIND THE FINGERPRINT OF DOOM?

Dr. Weinreb's mistake is relevant to our current understanding of the brain and dementia. Instead of fingerprints on the hand, brain doctors now talk about finding the "fingerprints" of dementia or Alzheimer's disease in brain scans. Rather than reading the ink on a piece of paper, they are reading immensely expensive functional MRIs. But the results that they have for predicting dementia may not be any more accurate than what Dr. Weinreb found with his fingerprints.

Most of us know the basic model of Alzheimer's Disease involves amyloid plaques, these tangles of cells gone bad. Your doctor gets the MRI back, points to the scan, and tells you that you have plaques in your brain. Just like plaques on your teeth, these are bad news. The more plaques, the more damage, right?

Maybe.

Maybe not.

To get a sense of how confusing the state of diagnosing dementia and Alzheimer's disease has become, you need to know that there are old plaques and new plaques. Some researchers continue to argue that old plaques are the true cause of the problem. Other researchers have abandoned the old plaques and are arguing that the new plaques are the true issue.

THE OLD FINGERPRINT: AMYLOID PLAQUES

The old plaques were called amyloid plaques. They showed up in the brain that Alois Alzheimer sliced open back in 1906 (the patient had passed on) and provided a clear sign of dementia. But the old plaques don't show any direct connection to how bad the Alzheimer's disease becomes.

I know, that's disturbing, because all these years we've been thinking, "more plaques equal more disease." It makes logical sense,. Everyone agreed. It was the basis for all treatment ideas right up to ten years ago.

But it's not true.[xxvii]

There are older people with lots of amyloid plaques who look like they should have advanced Alzheimer's disease but who are living normal lives. And there are people who have relatively few plaques, with healthy-looking brains, who cannot remember their names.

Don't believe me. Believe the expert researchers who have dedicated their lives to finding the connection. "For many years, investigators have been puzzled by the weak to nonexistent correlation between the amount of neuritic plaque pathology in the human brain and the degree of clinical dementia."[xxviii]

There's no direct relationship. But because the idea of amyloid plaques has been around for a long time, and there's been an enormous amount of money invested in following them, don't expect the amyloid plaque idea to go out of fashion any time soon.

THE NEW FINGERPRINT: TAU MARKERS

Now there is a new focus on tau markers. Why would we need new markers unless the amyloid plaque model no longer worked? But the argument is that the tau markers, which are generated by degenerating brain tissue, are just a better, more specific measure of brain loss than the older, more general amyloid plaques. In other words, the amyloid plaques are the result of general brain breakdown; the tau markers are how much is breaking down right this second. Tau markers are the new, improved version of the plaque model of memory loss.

So how well do the tau markers predict the advance of Alzheimer's disease or dementia?

Let's put the numbers in context.

Remember the numbers given by Dr. Weinreb? He thought his fingerprints gave 83% sensitivity and 63% specificity.

The current tau markers, the forefront of our extremely expensive and complex new brain lab technology for predicting memory loss, give "sensitivity...from 51% to 90% ...specificity ...from 48% to 88%." If that sounds like tau markers are questionable, let's take the researchers' own word for it. "The insufficiency and heterogeneity of research...leads to a state of uncertainty regarding the value of CSF testing."[xxix]

Remember, these tau marker experiments are only single-blind experiments. These researchers are trying to find a connection by staring at brain scans of patients they know have dementia. Like Dr. Weinreb, they know what they're looking for, but they still can't find any good connection. So the connection between the brain scans and dementia is weaker than the connection between our fingerprints and dementia. At this point, we might be better off just looking at people's hands. It would be cheaper and just as accurate.

BUT SHOULDN'T WE RUN THE TESTS ANYWAY?

Now, the argument your doctor would make is that there isn't any harm in testing for either amyloid plaques or these new tau markers. After all, what harm could it do? Shouldn't we find out if the tests are positive?

But the researchers know exactly how much damage can be caused by using questionable markers to decide if your memory loss is due to Alzheimer's disease. "Particular attention should be paid to the risk of misdiagnosis and overdiagnosis of dementia (and therefore over-treatment) in clinical practice."[xxx]

Take it from someone who spent decades being afraid of his fingerprints.

We don't have definitive proof that plaques of any kind cause memory loss, and we know for certain that more plaques don't equal a worse diagnosis. So doctors need to base their treatment on patient symptoms rather than what's showing up on the screen. And a reasonable argument could be made that testing for Alzheimer's is likely to cause harm and anxiety without providing significant benefit.

So if more amyloid plaques and tau markers don't cause Alzheimer's disease and dementia, what does cause it in the brain?

We don't know.

The reality is that we're probably talking about many different diseases, not one or two. We're still trying to classify memory loss by what we can see in a scan or in a lab when neither one gives us a clear picture of what's going on. By combining many different types of dementia based on what we see in the lab we're making our ability to deal with memory loss impossibly complicated. We need to start back at square one to isolate the true causes of memory loss and then rename the diseases based on what will help people minimize their memory loss.

7 Memory Loss, Now What?

Annual mandatory screening for memory loss isn't a popular idea, because we don't have good treatments. As you get older, word tends to get around that it doesn't do any good to get the dementia diagnosis, and it might increase your insurance costs. One study found that half of those older adults who screened positive for memory loss refused follow up diagnostic testing.[xxxi] They'd rather not know.

WHAT HAPPENS IF YOU TEST POSITIVE?

Once you test positive for MCI, you become eligible for treatment. A range of drugs is available. All hold memory-creating chemicals in the brain longer, so they help a little with short term memory. As recently as 2015 doctors were arguing that they might have some longer term effect on memory loss.[xxxii]

But other researchers have asked questions about why the patients in the memory drug trials are significantly younger (more than five years) than the average dementia patient.[xxxiii] Five years difference alters the expected rate of dementia and younger patients would be expected to have less severe dementia.

How well do the drugs work?

Not well.

In January of 2018 an exhaustive review of all the studies (142) found that the memory drugs alone or in combination "have minimal effects on cognition."[xxxiv] For decades researchers have suspected this is the case[xxxv] and also been concerned about the side effects and drug interactions of these drugs. In 2012, a French medical journal advised against the use of the drugs because they likely did more harm than good. Finally in 2018 the French National Authority For Health (HAS) delisted the drugs for health care coverage, saying the drugs had "nothing to offer" dementia patients and could hasten death.[xxxvi] Meanwhile, other experts are still trying to standardize the best doses of the drugs for different stages of dementia.[xxxvii] So being eligible to receive drug treatment for dementia is definitely something to discuss with your doctor rather than to just start taking.

If you are screened and test positive for advanced memory loss, your living situation can have major effects on your long term health.

How that situation changes is due to several factors. The first factor is your family. Your family often determines how you'll be treated. In a family situation where you have a caregiver, the caregiver will most often make your decisions for you. If that person does not consider your memory loss a problem, then - regardless of the screening and diagnosis- you may stay right where you are and still be at the same risks.[xxxviii] In some cases, training your caregiver to give you better care can be as effective as treating you directly.[xxxix] The second factor is how involved your doctor is in changing your situation.[xl] So the attitude of your caregiver and your doctor are likely to be more of a factor for your care than whether or not you have a positive screening for memory loss.

If we are diagnosed with memory loss, is there anything we can do? Can we at least slow memory loss? I think it's possible. It won't be easy, but we can get there. Let's look at some of the causes of memory loss to figure out what we can do.

8 What Are Memories and How Are They Lost?

The memory loss we care about is that loss that happens during dementia. Unfortunately, we can only make some simple generalizations about memory. But those generalizations can help us find out how to keep the memories we want.

We're all forgetting all the time. Our sense memories last about half a second.[xli] Right now, your body is in a posture. In a few minutes, you may shift your body. You will instantly forget how that first posture felt, focusing on the new posture. Only now that I've brought it to your attention are you likely to even notice how fast you're forgetting. Remember what you ate today? How about last week? How did the food today compare to the same food you ate a month ago? A year? Was the clothing you wore yesterday softer than the clothing you're wearing today? We don't remember 99% of our lives. It's only the 1% we want to keep with us.

Should we try for more than 1%? Probably not.

There are very rare people who hang onto more than 1%. They are labelled as perfect recall subjects, but their ability to remember every day, every encounter, and the weather on that day doesn't seem to help them that much in life. In further analysis, they are so good at recalling the weather because they spend a lot of time recalling the weather. For other memory tests, they are just average. All the things they do recall come with a lot of anxiety rather than pleasure. It's more of an obsessive need to hold onto the past than a memory goal we should all aspire to accomplish.[xlii] So the 1% most of us remember is likely just enough, as long as we keep it.

How do you lose the memories you care about?

SHORT TERM MEMORY

The first memories you lose that you care about are your short-term memories. These are the memories you use to hold things for a few minutes and you don't mind forgetting in a few minutes later. Like why you came into the kitchen, or what you were going to do with that piece of cheese. The reason these things are easy to forget is that:

1) they aren't that important, and
2) we're easily distracted.

Any and all health concerns can also disrupt short-term memory. Poor sleep, hunger, background noise, bumping your toe, any of these can be responsible for short-term memory loss. So anyone, at any age, can have short-term memory loss. It's only concerning when it gets to be really bad.

LONG TERM MEMORY

Long term memory is much, much larger than short-term memory. Think of it like how much music your phone can store vs. how many songs you can play at one time. You can store thousands of songs/memories, but your short-term memory can only play one of those songs at any one time. So the simplest trick to increase your memory is to convert your lists and simple daily chores from short-term to long-term memory. You can do this by actively trying to remember them, making them more vivid, bizarre, or colorful. It really doesn't matter what technique you use, because your short-term memory is being set up somewhere in the longer term memory.

CONVERTING SHORT TO LONG TERM:

USE YOUR HOUSE

A simple way to attach short term memories to your long term memory is to visually put them into a known location. Take your house (any place you've lived long enough that you're familiar with every room) and your grocery list. Rather than trying to remember your grocery list by itself, take each item and put it into your home. The milk is in your bedroom, the eggs are in the hallway, the asparagus in the living room. Make them giant and moving, and you have your grocery list. When you get to the store, just walk through your house in your mind and pick up the wandering groceries as you go.

DIFFERENT PARTS OF LONG TERM MEMORY

Because long term memory is so big, we have to have lots of names for different types of long-term memory. I mention these not because there's a quiz later, but because dementia tends to affect the hippocampus of the brain. Some of these long-term memories rely on the hippocampus, and some don't. So it's really a good idea to understand that some of our memories may be more immune to memory loss from dementia.

ANYTHING TO DECLARE?

The two big groups of memory are declarative and implicit. I know, that means absolutely nothing. I could have defined them better as talking and silent. That might have been more helpful.

Declarative (talking) memory is the one we can talk about, recall at will and discuss.

Implicit (silent) memory is our memory of how to do things. Quick, describe how your nerves fire so you can lift your leg. Can't? No worries. Just lift your leg. You can't talk about it, but you can do it.

Just because we're getting into the memory weeds, now let's divide your declarative memory (talking) into episodic and semantic. In other words, my soap opera life vs. my quiz show life.

Our **episodic** memory is the soap opera of our life, all the traumatic or exciting things that ever happened to us. We don't try to remember every time we've ever had toast, just the one time the toaster caught on fire and almost burned the house down.

Our **semantic** (quiz show) memories are the facts that we think we know. The sun is bigger than the earth, I'm shorter than my brother, in the seventh grade I took social studies. These fact memories aren't emotional, just the facts.

THE WAY WE LOSE THESE MEMORIES ARE IN THE FOLLOWING ORDER:

First we lose our quiz show memories (semantic).

Then we lose our soap opera memories (episodic).

After all our conscious memories are gone, we still have our unconscious, silent, implicit memories. Why is that?

All of the declarative (talking) memories are processed by the hippocampus and have to be accessed by that one place in the brain. All of our implicit (silent) memories are stored in another place. So you can literally not be able to talk but still be able to drive. Or you can barely walk but still discuss philosophy. It depends on which areas of the brain are affected.

But remember, all memory was once implicit (silent). We learned to talk by hearing, wiggling our tongues, and figuring it out. So everything that becomes our declarative (talking) memory starts out as an implicit (silent) memory. It's got to go through the process of happening once before we can talk about it.

REPETITION EQUALS REMEMBERING

Once it becomes a talking memory, it can be made strong enough that you no longer need to do any memory recall. Something that you've remembered over and over again will become so set that you can remember it even if your "remembering equipment" in your brain no longer functions. I remember one of my patients who had almost no memory except one long, humorous story that she would start into every time someone looked at her. It was a good story the first time through. By the fifth or sixth time, it was pretty clear she was as frustrated as anyone else that the only thing she could remember was the one story. But it was in there, a perfectly preserved rose in a withered garden.

The destruction of the "remembering equipment" in the hippocampus prevents people from forming new memories. The old ones are still in there, especially the memories with strong connections to lots of different areas of your life. That's why people with dementia can still remember things from long ago, just nothing more recent.

WHAT STAYS AROUND LONGEST?

After the loss of short-term memories, the next thing that is likely to be lost is semantic (quiz show) memories. These are the dry facts and figures of life. How much was that cantaloupe? Who was the sixth president? Unless you have some connection emotionally to these things, they tend to drift away. (Hint: think of John Quincy Adams with his head like a cantaloupe with a giant six on it, and you might remember he was the sixth president. His dad was the second president.)

Words and language tend to go next. What is that thing called that you put on your head instead of real hair? Which is that long sounding color between pink and red? These are semantic (quiz show) issues, without any emotional color.

Next to go is our ability to remember how to get somewhere. Did you take Center Street to Lexington or Ninth? Was that little shop on this block or one block over? The rate of this directional loss is likely due to the original size of your hippocampus. It depends on whether you spend a lot of time learning the roads like an old-style London taxi driver (an ancient form of Uber or Lyft for the young readers). Today we never learn the roads at all, so electronic babysitting has taken this over for us completely.

Our life memories last the longest, with the most important holding the most connections. We fight for these memories just as we would if we were clinging to our scrapbooks coming out of a burning building.

What stays around the longest? Massive flashpoint memories. The Kennedy assassination. The moon landing. The fall of the

Berlin Wall. 9/11. These massive connection points remain even after our own lives have faded.

But we remember what we want to remember about these flashpoint days. Often our flashpoint memories, the ones we originally created about these days, weren't terribly accurate. It is that warped view of our life, where we'd like to have been on that fateful day, the conversation that never happened but that we remember so clearly, that we keep to the end.

9 What Causes 99% of Memory Loss?

If it's not genetics, almost all memory loss must be caused by diet and lifestyle. Right? That's the message of all the new memory recovery books. Just change your lifestyle and never lose your memories. They have some good suggestions we'll get to, but let's look at the big picture.

Does diet and lifestyle cause 99% of memory loss?

When we say 99%, it's not an exaggeration. The DIAN website says genetically-associated Alzheimer's disease affects less than 1%. So we really are talking about almost all memory loss being associated with diet and lifestyle. All we need to do is find out what causes memory loss and avoid it, yes? A lifetime of monk-like deprivation, no late nights or partying, but we'll be the Scrabble champs in the nursing home at the end.

The trouble is, we're not sure what kind of diet and lifestyle causes memory loss. If you dive into the different smaller studies about dementia risk, you can make yourself crazy. One study found most "common sense" issues like being a lonely couch potato with diabetes (and lots of other diseases) increased your dementia risk, except they found that smoking somehow lowered your risk.[xliii] Before you light up and start puffing away on your new pack-a-day health habit, another small study found that even passive, second-hand smoking increases your risk of developing dementia.[xliv] The results contradict each other, so it's hard to say what really causes dementia. Without any clear markers of what causes dementia, how can we know what to avoid?

Well, that's not true. We have one clear marker about what causes memory loss.

GETTING OLD

Don't get old. Or if you do get old, just make it to your eighties without memory loss. The only thing worse than getting old for developing memory loss is the alternative (but we're only guessing because no doctors have tested angels' memories in heaven).

GETTING REALLY SICK

We have an odd bump in memory loss between our fifties and our seventies. Coincidentally, we also have a big bump in deaths between our fifties and our seventies. There's also a bump in dementia between ninety and ninety-five. Which makes me wonder if we're just seeing seriously ill people and noting that their memory loss increases when they're really ill. I know my short-term memory was terrible when I was in the hospital for surgery. But that doesn't mean I had dementia, because I was as high as a kite and/or in a lot of pain. Anyone coming into my hospital room would not have gotten a clear picture of my non-pain mental state. She might have justifiably diagnosed me with MCI (minimal cognitive impairment), and if someone had scanned my brain and found a few plaques, I could be diagnosed with Alzheimer's disease right now. Rather than being far-fetched, this is an all-too-common situation as we get older.

Beyond aging, studies about lifestyle choices haven't been conclusive regarding memory loss. I've heard lots of strong ideas about what is definitely a cause, but researchers have tracked a lot of the common suspects for decades.

WHAT ELSE? THE BIG STUDIES

Rather than lose ourselves in the weeds of the small studies that argue for or against how bad some behavior is for memory, let's pick four big studies that track what causes memory loss over decades. These are called long abbreviations that researchers like, but which mean nothing to the rest of us.

The first is a **heart-based study**, where the researchers thought dementia was caused mostly by problems with the heart and blood vessels. It checked age, sex, education, blood pressure, weight, cholesterol, and exercise.

The second study was **brain-based**. Researchers figured that brain damage led to more brain damage and memory loss. The brain-based study checked age, education, weight, diabetes, stroke, needing assistance with money or medications, and depression.

The third study I'll call **the kitchen-sink** study. It went for the big picture, tracking everything but the kitchen sink. These researchers tracked age, sex, education, diabetes, traumatic brain injury, depression, brain exercises, cholesterol, social network, smoking, alcohol, exercise, weight, servings of fish, and pesticide exposure.

The fourth study is the **math-study**. Expert researchers in the math study tracked many of the same things as the other studies but used a very long, complicated, and impressive mathematical equation to calculate the risk of each thing on memory loss. In the equation they included age, sex, diabetes, weight, blood pressure, smoking, depression, stroke, aspirin use, and heart issues. So four studies, covering the heart, the brain, everything but the kitchen sink, and a mathematical equation all checked for lifestyle and dietary factors that affect memory loss.[xlv]

If you've made it through the last paragraph, hopefully you saw your own pet theory for what causes dementia mentioned. (I know a few of you will howl about heavy metals. We have no large studies.[xlvi]) After fifteen years of study, the winning model for predicting dementia is - drum roll please - none of the above. That's right, none of the studies from heart to the kitchen sink predicted whether or not a person would develop dementia better than a single, solitary marker.

Which single marker?

You guessed it.

Age.

Getting old told us as much about your risk of getting dementia as anything else. Nothing else made any major difference.

I know, it's hard to believe. As a lifelong researcher I'm suspicious that we're missing something with all this combining of things. I wrote this book thinking all I needed to do was tell people to be healthy and they'd be fine.

Another book to add to the pile of lifestyle books. "Healthy body, healthy mind," was what I thought I was going to be able to say. But we have to admit that it's pretty convincing when many independent researchers get together after decades of study and millions of research dollars and come to the same conclusion. They say "(A)ll models showed similar discriminative ability when compared to prediction based on age alone,"[xlvii] that means none of the other things made a big overall difference in dementia for the population as a whole.

SMALLER STUDIES

Now, you know I went looking for more information. "None of the above," doesn't fill a book even if you write it in really big letters.

You can reverse this no-effect on memory result by cherry picking out individual factors and looking at them for worsening dementia rates. Other researchers have done this for us. In a massive search of almost 17,000 medical articles, they identified 93 different factors in the medical literature that might affect memory (the kitchen sink study above only lists fifteen).

Of all the factors, the researchers then picked their top choices for what might benefit memory loss.

The researchers concluded that four drugs (estrogen, statins, blood pressure drugs, and aspirin) and four dietary supports (folate, vitamin C, vitamin E, and coffee) might help with dementia.

Keep in mind, they are literally cherry-picking for possible benefit. The larger studies above didn't find that these things made any difference. But some smaller studies did. So I'm including the information because I know people tend to "try things" anyway and I'd rather you did some vitamin C rather than desiccated weasel spleen or whatever they're selling you on your phone ads once the internet figures out you're interested in memory loss.

CHRONIC SICKNESS? MAYBE

When these look-for-anything researchers looked at medical conditions that affected memory loss, they found a much more complicated situation. Being weak, having high or low blood pressure, or having diabetes increased your risk of Alzheimer's disease. But having arthritis, heart disease, being just overweight, or having cancer decreased your risk of Alzheimer's disease. In looking at overall lifestyle, being fat or thin and not being educated increased your risk of Alzheimer's disease. In comparison, using your brain, smoking, drinking a little, being stressed, and being overweight decreased your risk of Alzheimer's disease.[xlviii]

For all of you who just felt good about being overweight, you're welcome. Same to those of you with vices like drinking or smoking who just felt validated. But remember, we're still not talking about significant differences in the overall population. All that was necessary to be included in this second huge search was a single study of any size. The really big, better studies of the overall population still say that none of the above will make a difference in the world's rate of dementia.

THE CAERPHILLY EFFECT

To get a real sense of how it's possible to have really good small studies that say certain things help but then have them contradicted by really big studies, I'd like to look at the Caerphilly study. Maybe it's just because I like the name, or maybe it's because they followed these patients for thirty years. The results they found were really good, and confirmed all my hopes for dementia.

Men who followed five healthy behaviors for thirty years had half as much death and two-thirds less dementia. What did they do? Simple things. Not smoking, drinking less than three drinks, walking four miles a day, eating three or more servings of vegetables and fruits, and keeping a normal body weight.

That's it. Do that for thirty years and you drop your risk of dementia by over 60%. But the trouble comes in when you start looking at the numbers.

They started with 2,235 men, but only 15 of those men ate four or more servings of fruits and vegetables. So to get their numbers up, they dropped the cutoff to three or more servings. But when they added up all the five behaviors, only 111 men did four of the five and only two did all five behaviors.

So when we say that doing all five behaviors dropped your risk of dementia, **we're talking about two guys**. Thank goodness one of them didn't get dementia, because otherwise the whole study would have been flipped on its head and we'd all be told to go drink and smoke, forget the exercise and vegetables. So you can have a really good, long term small study that doesn't really hold up when you want to expand it to the whole world's population.[xlix]

So it's not genetics, and it's not big obvious things like smoking, weight, heart disease, etc. So what on earth really causes memory loss?

10 Is It Use It Or Lose It?

We have a model for the rest of the body that seems to work. A muscle is weak, so we exercise it. As we put it under pressure, that muscle responds by getting stronger. Could it be the same for the brain?

Even as late at 2013, the studies on use it or lose it for memory function said "don't bother."[l] But with the utter failure of medications to affect long term memory loss, there's been an explosion in interest in alternatives. Of all the studies on memory exercises researchers looked at in 2017, 92% of them had been done recently. And the recent studies found much more positive results.[li]

SHORT TERM? YES

Studies of memory exercises for dementia have always shown short term effects. They didn't show long term effects, so doing memory exercises a few times and then stopping didn't affect your overall memory or your chances of developing dementia. But these exercises continue to help short-term memory regardless of your stage of dementia. They should be mandatory.

A recent analysis showed that "memory-focused interventions effectively improved memory-related performance in people with cognitive disorders." That review was done in 2018, and claims to be "first comprehensive meta-analysis of special memory domains in people with cognitive disorders"[lii] It upsets me because it wasn't done decades before. Why did we wait so long to really look at something as simple as memory exercises for people with memory problems? If this were a traumatic brain injury, we'd at least give them a trial of rehabilitation before assigning them to just supportive care. We're just now discovering that the majority of dementia patients can, like traumatic brain injury patients, benefit from rehabilitation therapy?[liii]

THE PHYSICAL RESPONSE

Remember, these are short term effects. But rather than feeling down about that result, we should take it in stride. After all, if I do lots of leg lifts in my twenties, that doesn't mean my legs are going to be strong in my forties. Why would we think that memory exercises in my sixties would help me in my eighties?

In the same way, my leg lifts are not going to make my arms stronger. So after doing a lot of leg lifts I wouldn't be surprised that my arm strength hasn't improved. But again and again we see researchers upset that specific mental activities only strengthen those specific areas and don't help overall mental response. It's like they have patients do leg lifts and honestly expect their arms to get stronger as well.

Another ongoing frustration for researchers is whether or not we can grow new brain cells as we age. While the National Institutes of Health say it's probable that we do, they still think it's controversial if we truly can.[liv] But they're missing the point. It isn't whether we can build new neurons, it's whether we can change our brain cell connections and improve them as we age. Whether we can teach an old dog new tricks depends more on her ability to make new connections between her brain cells than on her ability to grow new ones. These type of changes, the growth of new connections between brain cells, are not controversial, and occur while other connections are lost.[lv] They are recognized to exist at any age by all researchers.[lvi]

WHAT IF YOU'VE LOST IT?

But, you might say, doesn't it matter how many brain cells I have? Not really. Sure, if you're missing half of your brain it can impact you.[lvii] By impact, I mean it can make things difficult, not impossible. We have a documented case of a young woman who graduated high school while missing the entire left side of her brain since birth.[lviii]

Anything short of missing half your brain can be bad, but distant portions of your brain can rewire themselves to help you cope.[lix] The key is that the brain is very changeable, even throughout our adulthood. In her bestselling memoir *My Stroke of Insight*, neuroanatomist Dr. Jill Bolte Taylor describes recovering from a massive left-sided stroke and continuing rehabilitation until she regains her mathematical ability eight years after the stroke.[lx] Her short TED talk on the subject is both remarkable and incredibly optimistic about our capacity to recover from brain injuries and overcome brain damage.[lxi]

So we know that memory loss is not genetic. It is not determined by a wide range of factors, many of which "should" impact memory. But memory loss is impacted dramatically by the use of memory. These changes are not long-term, they are short-term. And they are specific to the areas of the brain or the types of exercises done.

THE BRAIN AS A MUSCLE

At this point, the simplest way to think about your brain is to think about it the same way as your arm muscles. It will make the rest of the book much easier to understand.

When I was a high-school freshman, I broke my left arm in a spectacular fall over a soccer ball. This was still in the age when they casted arms for extended periods. My left arm was in a cast for three months. When the cast came off, my left arm could barely move. The muscle had atrophied. Don't worry, they told me, it will come back.

My left arm did come back, but it wasn't because of my genetics or a lifestyle factor like eating more cheese. None of possible causes mentioned for memory loss would apply to my left arm either.

I needed to focus on the specific deficits in my arm and work every day to make them stronger. As part of my recovery, I realized that my arm was bent funny, and I needed to lift things a little differently with that arm. So every day I worked with my arm to help it get back to where my left arm and my right arm are now nearly equal.

THE NOCEBO EFFECT

Here's what didn't happen during my left arm recovery. No white-coated doctor told me that my arm might never recover. No one explained to me that some loss of function was to be expected as I aged, and no one showed me high tech images of a functional MRI of my withered left arm and explained that the muscle loss was likely permanent.

Can you imagine what I might have done as a high school student if they had? At that point, without a medical degree of my own, I would have believed them. I wouldn't try to heal my arm, just learn to strap it to my side and do it all with my right. Over time the arm atrophy would continue and worsen. They might even recommend a surgery to remove my now useless arm to make my life easier.

Thank goodness we don't treat arms the way we treat minds. We lack any evidence that physical testing of the brain directly applies to memory loss. But doctors are using inaccurate laboratory testing and bad screening to justify telling patients that nothing can be done. These are caring practitioners who want the best outcomes for patients. But their assessments only address a snapshot of what is happening right now rather than what could be happening in the future with aggressive rehabilitation.

If I came into a doctor's office with memory loss and underwent testing, chances are good that I would show some memory loss on the tests. Depending on the doctor, that memory loss would be seen as either minimal or as a sign of greater deterioration to come. In no case would the doctor give me any better news than, "You're not losing your mind, yet." Without treatments, those with worse diagnoses are simply sent home to get their affairs in order before they lose their minds. No one is being given the choice of rehabilitation regardless of their condition.

Maybe continued memory loss is the likely outcome, but I know that the most likely outcomes are a result of not taking any action to avoid them. Just as my arm would not have improved without specific interventions, minds do not improve without daily effort.

BETTER THAN ARM MUSCLES

But, some of you are asking, isn't there a point of no return? A point at which nothing can be done? Maybe. But I know that after a stroke patients are given rehabilitation treatment up to a year. Neuroanatomist Dr. Taylor got results after eight years of rehabilitation. So I don't think we've even started to explore the ability of the mind to recover.

But most of us don't wait a decade to take action if our arm is hurting. We know that a very short period of inactivity can cause a loss of strength. One estimate is that a bed rest of five weeks will drop your physical strength in half.[lxii] That's a use it or lose it call to action.

By comparison, mental inactivity doesn't result in as rapid a complete loss of function. But anyone who has learned a foreign language knows that not using it over a period of time makes it "rusty." What is remarkable is how fast the language (the brain connections) return once you start using the language again. It would be like having five weeks of bed rest and returning to full strength within a day or two. The brain is remarkably responsive.

Let's end with the story of a harpsichord player who could not recognize the word "thumb" and had no idea what a corkscrew was. But when he was placed with his instrument, he could play beautifully. More amazing, he could play any new pieces placed before him. The areas of his brain for music were so well developed they outlasted almost everything but breathe itself.[lxiii] Our goal is to strengthen our areas of vital living so they continue long after their expected deterioration.

11 Removing The Obstacles

When you look for cures for Alzheimer's disease you come across very excited articles claiming to reverse Alzheimer's when the true cause was another disease.[lxiv] A whole host of other diseases can cause memory problems. One of the people promoting this as a cure for dementia is Dr. Bredesen, who has received coverage from medical journals.[lxv]

Dr. Dale E. Bredesen has a fascinating book called *The End Of Alzheimer's* which is a hopelessly optimistic title, but I admire his confidence. What Dr. Bredesen is really doing in his book is listing out a plan for systematically getting rid of all the other possible common causes of memory loss besides dementia. He doesn't treat dementia so much as treat around it.

To make my point clear, if I wrote a book called *The End of Pain* and then wrote about how I'd noticed that many patients with pain had badgers attacking their legs. These badgers did cause a lot of leg pain, and removing the badgers would really benefit some people. But in no way would badger removal be the end of all pain. If you had badger pain, it would be great. But if you didn't have any badger attacking your legs, my badger removal strategies wouldn't help you at all.

Given that the title of his book claims the impossible, I went to what Dr. Bredesen has published in the medical journals. In 2014 he published a study of ten patients he ran through his program.

His results were nothing less than miraculous. Nine of the ten showed either subjective or objective improvements. Six of them had been working before their memory loss and were able to go back to their jobs.

These are very impressive results compared to the standard medical reality of gradual memory decline. Dr. Bredesen writes very movingly in his book about several of his patients, describing how one had decided suicide was preferable to following in her mother's footsteps into dementia. But however moving, we have to keep in mind the Caerphilly effect, the idea that a few people getting better doesn't mean that everyone will benefit.

REDISCOVERING OLD SCHOOL MEDICINE

What struck me about Dr. Bredesen's approach was how closely it follows what I consider to the basis of Naturopathic medicine. For those of you who aren't familiar with it, Naturopathic medicine is a highly individualized medical model that attempts to identify the cause of an illness rather than manage symptoms. We spend a great deal of time with each patient, learning what specific diet or lifestyle factors may be most impacting them. Then we create a treatment plan based on their needs rather than a standardized plan.

In 2014 Dr. Bredesen's treatment of his patients lists a large number of interventions.[lxvi]

They range from the common sense: get enough sleep, exercise regularly, do brain exercises, and reduce stress. I'm on board with this for every patient.

Dr. Bredesen adds a large number of supplements: coconut oil, resveratrol, B vitamins, Selenium, CoQ10, vitamin C, Omega 3s, Vitamin E, Vitamin D, and NAC. He also adds in a number of herbs: Gotu kolu, turmeric, Ashwaghanda, and Lion's Mane mushroom.

Then Dr. Bredesen looks for other common diseases that can cause dementia as a side effect. Thyroid or other hormonal balances are checked in every patient. Homocysteine levels and insulin levels are brought down. If there is sleep apnea (when you stop breathing during sleep), that is treated. If there are vitamin deficiencies, those are brought to an optimal level. In the end, most people on Dr. Bredesen's plan feel better about their brain and some even have a measurable improvement on the tests.

If Dr. Bredesen's plan feels like a cocktail of different treatments, that's because it is. He's been researching HIV patients since the 1980s and in 2013 decided that another route was needed for Alzheimer's disease. Dr. Bredesen literally wrote that "the optimal therapeutic approach to AD does indeed turn out to involve a multi-component cocktail"[lxvii] and he is continually looking for more things to make up that cocktail.

HOW WELL DOES IT WORK?

We need to think for a moment about Dr. Bredesen's numbers. In 2014 he's treating ten patients and not all of them got better. After intense intervention, one of the patients did not improve. Of the patients who did get better, not all of them had testable improvements. But Dr. Bredesen used these results to publish his book. That's a lot of weight to hang on a few patient success stories.

If you follow along with Dr. Bredesen over the past few years, of the first 125 patients he's had go through his program, 50% saw improvement. The best outcomes he's had are with early memory loss.[lxviii] At this point, no other researchers have repeated his program, so we're depending entirely on his results.

If this reminds you at all of Dr. Weinreb and his fingerprints, that's what concerns me. I've read through dozens of less famous medical journal articles by doctors convinced the causes of dementia are environmental, genetic, infectious, or societal. They all make convincing arguments and can point to small studies that support their point of view. But none of them are claiming that they've found the cure. Dr. Bredesen may share Dr. Weinreb's strong medical pedigree and his confidence. I pray he does not share Dr. Weinreb's mistaken assumptions.

ADDING TO THE LIST

Dr. Bredesen does not mention anything about mold exposure

in his initial assessment in 2014, but he adds it in 2015. He calls it inhalational Alzheimer's disease, and it makes up one of the three types of Alzheimer's he feels are distinctly different diseases.[lxix] These three Dr. Bredesen writes about as inflammatory, non-inflammatory, and early onset. Initially he thought the early onset form was at least partially due to a zinc deficiency.[lxx] Now it's due to mold exposure. We are seeing Dr. Bredesen's Alzheimer's cocktail evolve as he works to improve his results. So far, he's the only researcher who's done his work, with only one other medical citation that even discusses his plan.[lxxi]

ASSUME HE'S RIGHT

What if Dr. Bredesen is right. He has found the cure for Alzheimer's? If so, why does his current model only help half the patients? Still, half is better than none. And he's constantly tweaking his list to improve his results. So we should be seeing his plan roll out across the U.S., right? Not likely.

Let me be perfectly clear. I absolutely applaud Dr. Bredesen's plan, his dedication, and his ability to see the need for an entirely new treatment model. His ideas are from the AIDs population, which embraced alternatives and supportive treatments long before integrative medicine was even a real idea.

I was brought up with those integrative ideas, I practice them every day. When I read through what Dr. Bredesen is doing, I am familiar with every aspect of his protocol. So I am absolutely the right person to say that Dr. Bredesen's program will not work for the population as a whole.

For individuals, Dr. Bredesen's program will give results. If you have any minor memory loss, following just the commonsense aspects of eating right, getting enough sleep and reducing your stress are likely to improve your memory. I'm not as sold on the whole plan.

A typical basic plan for Dr. Bredesen would look something like this:

1. eliminating all simple carbohydrates, gluten and processed food from the diet, and eating more

vegetables, fruits and non-farmed fish
2. meditating twice a day and beginning yoga to reduce stress
3. sleeping seven to eight hours per night, up from four to five
4. taking melatonin, methylcobalamin, vitamin D3, fish oil and coenzyme Q10 each day
5. optimizing oral hygiene using an electric flosser and electric toothbrush
6. reinstating hormone replacement therapy, which had previously been discontinued
7. fasting for a minimum of 12 hours between dinner and breakfast, and for a minimum of three hours between dinner and bedtime
8. exercising for a minimum of 30 minutes, four to six days per week[lxxii]

How well did his patients follow their plans? They didn't. Dr. Bredesen admitted that none of his patients followed his entire plan for them.

Dr. Bredesen's hope is that he can spark enough interest to generate funding for a large, double-blind trial of his treatment plan. He used reports from across the country to show that different doctors can use his approach to improve the lives of individual patients. In a hundred patient reports, many showed some improvement, and a few showed tremendous improvement.[lxxiii]

IS IT FOR EVERYONE?

But the system that Dr. Bredesen wants to put into place is not scalable. It is not a solution for the population as a whole, and I say this as someone who dearly wishes it was. Most people do not want to dramatically change their lifestyles to get well. Of those that do, few can afford a cupful of supplements every day. Even fewer can afford the extensive testing that Dr. Bredesen requires to find out what else might ail them. Of those, only the wealthy could afford to fully treat those other conditions once he includes things like mold exposure.

I wish it was just a matter of money. In Washington state, Naturopathic medicine is covered by insurance. So the tests and the visits to doctors like Dr. Bredesen are covered in that state. But fewer than 3% of patients seek out and follow that intensive model of medicine.[lxxiv] We are too well trained as a population to look for a drug or a surgical solution to think that diet and lifestyle will truly reverse our chronic illnesses.

MEDICAL INERTIA

There is a prejudice against lifestyle medicine within modern medicine. It is fueled in part by a focus on acute, ER style medicine, where lifestyle change is too slow to make a difference.

But it is also fueled by an aggressive skeptical community that sees anything alternative as immediately suspect and threatening to scientific medicine. They unwittingly play into the hands of the pharmaceutical industry, who are happy to publicize the failures of herbs or lifestyle while minimizing the side effects of the drugs they sell.

I don't think of this as a conspiracy, simply the medical version of the culture wars and a need to maintain market share. But that internal medical prejudice will ensure that Dr. Bredesen's plan will never get the true test it needs to see how effective it could be.

Instead, we should look for aggressive marketing of his supplements, and possibly the extraction and patenting of anything he finds truly helpful. Look for a new drug for dementia patients, not the creation of clinics.

I don't want to sound pessimistic, just realistic. Dementia care is set to become a trillion dollar industry in the next thirty years. Nursing homes and all the staff needed to fill them will be a growth sector. Anything that threatens that growth sector is likely to be suspect. Particularly anything that cannot be patented and sold at a premium.

WILL A MAJOR STUDY CHANGE IT?

To even give Dr. Bredesen's plan traction, a large-scale clinical trial would need to be done. It would need to have fairly miraculous results, and I would love to see those results prove him correct. But it would still likely be relegated to the sidelines of the dementia treatment model.

If Dr. Bredesen's program did pass clinical trials, what would we get? Not the kind of change we'd like to see.

We have our example in the amazing work of Dr. Dean Ornish. Dr. Ornish showed he could reverse heart disease using a multi-disciplinary approach similar in many ways to Dr. Bredesen's work. Dr. Ornish's results were robust, and the cost savings show that it's half as expensive to put heart patients through the Ornish program than into standard heart care.[lxxv]

The Ornish program is now covered by medicare, which means that people are falling over themselves to enroll for this proven treatment, right?

No.

Out of a possible 3,600 eligible patients, only 140 enrolled in Ornish's program. Another 440 selected a less intense program. The rest chose the more expensive, more risky, standard care. If you do the math, not quite 4% of eligible patients chose a lifestyle program that was proven to lower their heart attack risk.[lxxvi]

So I'm not being pessimistic about Dr. Bredesen's program. I wish him the greatest success. But I also know that the culture of medicine he's working within has an amazing inertia towards easy solutions regardless of clinical outcomes. We expect a drug or surgery even when lifestyle is proven to be better treatment.

WHAT DOES THAT MEAN FOR YOU?

But we're not worried about the population as a whole in this book. For you, dear reader, the goal is to improve your own memory. To do that, do make sure you aren't currently suffering from a vitamin deficiency or another disease. Take particular care to watch for diabetes, low thyroid, and sleep apnea. If any of these areas have not been checked for you or a loved one with dementia, I urge you to aggressively pursue diagnosis and treatment. I've seen miraculous recoveries when other diseases heal and ease the burden on the brain.

There's also an area that Dr. Bredesen misses. Polypharmacy, the over prescribing of unnecessary medications to people with memory loss. Some studies of medication overuse found that over half of patients with dementia were overmedicated.[lxxvii] Another study of antipsychotic medications found that the medications could increase the rate of death for patients with dementia.[lxxviii]

We'll go through Dr. Bredesen's different herbs a bit later, with the goal that you will eat as food anything that may be helpful. Not because supplements are ineffective, but because most people stop their supplements within two years. If we want long-term change it needs to be food. Unless humanity changes a great deal, you'll still be eating food a decade from now.

And please, don't assume that your memory is your primary problem. If you're not sleeping, if you've been burning the candle at both ends, or if you never move your body, all of these can have secondary memory loss. Continuing to do these behaviors means all the brain exercises in the world won't solve your problem.

12 What Should We Eat?

Remember, nothing you eat will save your memory. So this should be a short chapter, right? But many things that you eat can help your brain work better today. Let's talk about food generally and then get specific about what will help you remember today, tomorrow, and next week. Who knows? Maybe you can prove the big studies are wrong in your case.

MEMORY ENERGY

The brain uses a lot of energy to think. About 20% of your total body energy goes to your head on a given day. That's a lot of calories, and the brain uses only two kinds of fuel. The first we all know, sugar. The second is less familiar unless you have been on an Atkins-style diet: ketones.

Let's talk about sugar first. If you eat sugar, your blood sugar rises. That's why a sugary snack can sometimes help you think better for the next few minutes. The key is that the same sugar is going to trigger off a burst of insulin, which is going to bring down your blood sugar and make you sleepier in another hour. So that donut for the morning meeting likely means you get twenty minutes of focused time and an hour of drowsy inattention.

A much better plan is to use a variety of fuels to help your brain function in both the short term and long term. You want your brain to be able to burn fuel all day long, like a furnace or a campfire.

Straight sugar is like kindling, it burns fast, but it burns out. Sure, you can keep adding kindling, but eventually it's going to run out. Adding protein or fats is like adding larger logs to a campfire. They don't burn as fast, but they burn a lot longer. So combining them with any sugar will give you less of an initial bump but a much longer burn. Instead of twenty minutes of focus and an hour of inattention, you'll get a whole meeting where you can focus enough not to lose your job.

SIMPLE IS BETTER

OK, so we know we need a variety of fuels. Which ones? Think simple, think nutritional labels you can understand. If you pick up a potato, the ingredients would say, "contains: potato." If you pick up a bag of potato chips, the ingredients can go as long as your arm. What's wrong with that?

Let me introduce you to "subclinical hepatic encephalopathy." [lxxix] What? Think hangover. Any time a person decides to drink they can develop a hangover. It's a combination of dehydration and the buildup of alcohol's breakdown products in their blood. These break down products circulate, and some of them get up into the brain, slowing its processing and inflaming the brain lining. People who are hung over have subclinical hepatic encephal-opathy, a backup of material the liver hasn't been able to process yet. You don't want them in charge of delicate operations or doing the math for a moon landing in that state.

But what does alcohol have to do with potato chips (other than they go well together)? Plenty. All of those compounds added to your humble potato need the liver to break them down. Get enough of those long word chemicals in your body, and you can back up the liver. In other words, you can get a low grade hangover from processed food. All the side effects without the buzz. That doesn't mean you can't eat them, and some of us have faster livers than others so we don't even notice the effects. But why would you add a possible hangover when it wasn't fun to get there? So keep your food choices simple, which simplifies your liver's job and lessens your chance of having fuzzy brain from some additive.

THE ITALIANS GOT IT RIGHT

Right, simple food? Which ones?

In a word, Mediterranean.

What? Come on, you know the drill. Good fats (olive oil), lots of vegetables, little red meat, some fish, whole grain brown carbs, only a little sugar, drink alcohol with dinner only, and don't smoke.

Small studies putting patients with dementia on Mediterranean diets show improved brain function after four years.[lxxx],[lxxxi]

Why? It has less to do with the olive oil base, the salads, the meat as condiment, and the focus on whole foods. The biggest thing is that a Mediterranean diet done right forces you to eat slowly, with friends, and enjoy your food. Think of it as the opposite of horking your six month old "power bar" in your car while careening from work to the first of three evening parties. That's not food, that's barely survival.

Food should be smelled before it's tasted. It should be fletcherized (that's chewed enough that you don't choke on every third bite). And it should be appreciated. Think of your meals as the sensory equivalent of a brain teaser. Name three other times you ate food that smelled this good. Tell one good joke you remember from one of those times. Do one toast to dear friends you recall from those times. See, food isn't a "get-through-it?" It's a use-it-or-lose-it for your senses.

WHAT ABOUT SUGAR?

If you have diabetes, controlling your blood sugar is a good idea for a host of reasons. But higher blood sugar does also seem to increase your risk of dementia in small studies. We're talking keeping your caramelized blood (Hb A1c) below 8%.[lxxxii] Beyond that, we don't have proof that sugar does much.

What?

I know, it seems like we should have more proof that high sugar levels do more damage. Major medical journals report things like dementia is caused by: "risk factors of high BMI, high fasting plasma glucose, smoking, and a high intake of sugar-sweetened beverages."[lxxxiii] But that study also only reported that one third of dementia was preventable, so I'm not sure where they're getting their information.

The last point about sugary soda is a little specific. If you want to go down that rabbit hole, there are researchers who argue that soda destroys sleep, hurts babies, makes you clumsy, causes ADHD,[lxxxiv] and makes you hate God. Well, I made up that last one, but I think if I asked them they might agree. Maybe they have a point, but there's still dementia in places where they can't afford soda. I think we can lose focus on the bigger picture by focusing too much on what soda does to rats.

WHAT ABOUT MEAT?

After my colon cancer I went from a "just one" dieter to "none for me" person. That's vegan, gluten-free, and sugar-free. Yes, I'm still working on my very short cookbook.

But that doesn't mean doing any of those things is going to help with dementia. There are some concerns about B12 and dementia, but few vegans miss their supplements. Can we get a verdict on meat and dementia?

A study out of California estimated that eating meat doubled your chances of dementia, but only in one group in the study. The other group didn't see any difference.[lxxxv] Any major difference between vegetarians and meat eaters is likely to be due to vegetarians having less heart disease rather than a decreased rate of dementia itself.[lxxxvi] In other words, the vegan doctor is telling you that you can still eat meat.

SHOULD WE NOT EAT LIKE THE FINNISH?

If you've been sifting through the world dementia data (now that's a thrill-filled afternoon) you might find that Finland has the highest rate of dementia in the world.

Why?

Is it the Finnish diet?

Not likely. The Finns eat relatively well. They are actually rated overall as one of the healthiest countries by Forbes.[lxxxvii] One of the reasons for that ranking is that the Finns have one of the highest life expectancy rates for men. Older men mean higher rates of dementia. It's a byproduct of their successful national healthcare system.

But that doesn't stop researchers from looking for more nefarious reasons for their dementia rates, including a high concentration of bacteria in their water that can cause dementia. [lxxxviii] This despite the Finns scoring very high on environmental standards.

My favorite reason for the increased dementia rate in Finland is that the Finns are moving away from their traditional sauna lifestyle. In another small study, the rate of dementia dropped among Finns based on the number of saunas they did every week.[lxxxix] To the saunas!

WHAT'S THE POINT?

The point is that you can get very confused and misled by small studies, ending up following terrible or extreme advice based on the outcomes of thirteen Eskimos or an odd group of twenty-seven Californians who eat only while hanging upside down. Please don't let someone sell you on a major lifestyle change without a lot of questions.

At the same time, there is good reason for thinking about improving your lifestyle and diet. While we have big studies that didn't find much difference, we may have missed the forest for the trees. As one researcher put it,

"Total midlife healthy dietary changes (improving quality of fats, increasing vegetables, decreasing sugar and salt) were associated with a reduced risk of dementia…(by about half)…In contrast, when each factor was assessed individually, associations were not significant."[xc] The whole lifestyle and diet change may be greater than the sum of its parts.

What if we're wrong? "A healthy lifestyle with daily outdoor activity and a Mediterranean diet not only reduces the risk of dementia, but also of coronary death and cancer."[xci] If we're wrong, we don't die of other things. That's not a bad trade off. Pass the olive oil.

13 How Should We Exercise?

Move it or lose it.

Does this mean you should exercise?

Yes, you should walk an hour a day. No more, no less. Why? Because walking an hour a day sets up an inflammation/heal response in the human body. It may not directly affect your brain, but it's a good start.

But physical exercise alone will not save your memory. It helps avoid memory loss due to things like heart attacks or strokes, but it's not a direct helper.

Next, we need to exercise our brains.

The bottom line is that you need to upgrade your brain. Bring things from one level of memory to the next level to increase your memory of them.

ONE: IF YOU DON'T COMMIT IT TO MEMORY, IT DOESN'T COUNT.

If you've ever been at a party, and introductions are flying, there are names you don't even catch on the first go around. It was Marcie, Chad, mumble, and Greg. Unless you ask mumble for her name again, no fair thinking you're losing your mind if you don't remember mumble's name in the supermarket six weeks later.

When we're young, we understand this truth. As we get older, the mumbles of the world get under our skin in a way we shouldn't let them.

The same thing applies to my grocery list. It constants changes. I do not commit it to memory. The simple reality is that as I'm driving around the supermarket I'll remember things that weren't on the grocery list. Oh, we needed this or that, some of the other. So at the end I'll look at the picture I took of the grocery list and make sure I've gotten all those items as well. But if you asked me what was on my grocery list, or told me that kumquats were on there, I'd be hard pressed to say you were wrong. No, I don't remember us ever eating kumquats (voluntarily), but I have no idea what's on that list.

I'm also the king of random trivia. Rainfall in Zimbabwe? I might know that. Metric weight of a muskrat? It's possible that number is rattling around in there somewhere. I know I remember blood pressures and birthdays of some of my patients. But none of that has been committed to memory. That's all "memory leaves" that have blown in and parked themselves in some corner of my brain. Maybe it's in there, and maybe not. But I don't expect it to be in there, and I'm not going to lose my mind over whether I'm losing my mind if I don't remember the number of children Bach had (twenty or twenty-one, he was a busy man).

TWO: DON'T PRETEND YOU CAN REMEMBER PAST THINGS IF YOU'RE STRESSING NOW.

Adrenaline is great for when you're trying to remember a current situation.[xcii] Skydiving? Going to remember that. Running from wolves? Pretty good chance that will stick in the ol' memory banks.

But try doing a geography test after running from wolves or skydiving. The same stress hormones that will help you remember a traumatic incident will also block your ability to remember all the random flotsam you stored away months ago. This isn't an age thing, though as we age we often use more effort to remember things (more in there to remember, and fewer connections). Even young healthy volunteers are unable to remember test answers when they're stressed.[xciii]

It makes sense if you think about it. The body was set up to do one set of things when really stressed. Fight or flight. The blood is put out to your arms and legs to get you ready to do either one. That leaves a lot less blood to go hunting for the capital of Hungary (Budapest, but I looked it up to make sure). So a stress response is the opposite of a remembering response. For that you need to rest and digest. You need that after-dinner warm glow where you sit around reminiscing about your glory days.

The problem is that if you're stressed about remembering, you're less likely to remember. Better to assume a worse memory than you have, be excited when you do remember things, and give yourself a break for the rest of the time. It's going to take the edge off, give you more brain blood flow, and ultimately help you remember things better.

THREE: DO STRESS NOW ABOUT REMEMBERING THE THINGS YOU WANT TO REMEMBER NOW.

Your kids' names. Your combination to your safe. Your important numbers. When there's something really important you need to remember, adding stress to that memory is going to bring it into high relief for you.

THE STEPS TO REMEMBERING

The way we forget is the way to remember.
Short-term memory is the key.
It's like the number of things you can run on an old computer before the computer slows way down. Or the number of things you can do on your phone while it's updating itself. Maintaining and engaging short-term memory means transferring anything unnecessary away from short-term memory space. Once that's done, you need to engage your short-term memory with a little bit of stress, an increased sense of the importance of the information you're trying to hold onto for a few minutes. Think of it as the "I'm a secret agent, this is the vital information necessary for the safety of the free world" memory booster. Remember those things

like your life depended on it. But just for a few minutes. Let go of the information afterward.

How do you free up your short-term memory? Convert anything else to long-term or muscle memory.

Long-term memory is vast. Making associations between the new material and something in your long-term memory is the key to retaining it longer. Think of it as figuring out the filing system in your head. You have one, it just puts old football scores next to memories of girls you once dated and those are right over the three recipes for meatloaf you still recall. It doesn't make sense to anyone but you. But that's not important. The important thing is to make those associations with something. Pick the number 9879 (I just made that up randomly). How do you want to remember that? I've got a bunch of ways.

One way I learned is to convert the number to letters, and then make words from the letters (I'll explain it in detail a bit later). If I remember the words, I can convert back to the number. It's complicated, and gets easier as you practice.

But let's assume you haven't learned any conversion system. Break down the numbers for yourself. Another way for me would be to look at 98 and 79. In 1998 I was just starting medical school. In 1979 I was in elementary school, but it's close enough to make me think about a new elementary school I had to start. So 9879 for me is a medical student and an elementary school student just starting out.. Once I convert that into an image of a doctor holding a nine-year-old's hand, I have a picture that means the same as that number.

Notice that I just spent some time trying to remember. It doesn't matter how I remember. Maybe for you that number is an old license plate, or the number of hot dogs you've eaten in your lifetime. The point is that engaging in the process of remembering is going to make that number convert out of your short-term memory into your long-term memory. If you do it right, at the end of this book you'll still remember the number even though while reading this book you've forgotten most of the more useful things I've said.

MUSCLE MEMORY

The other way to empty out your short-term memory is to convert much of what you do into muscle memory. What's muscle memory? It's easiest to talk about in a story.

You're driving down the highway. A song comes on. It reminds you of a spring day when you were young. For the length of the song you're transported away to another year, a vivid set of memories. The song ends and you "come back." Where were you? Memoryland. But why didn't you die in a screaming wreck on the side of the road? Muscle memory.

All the time your conscious brain was remembering, your body was still remembering how to drive. Your reflexes coordinated with your eyes, your feet monitored your speed, and you kept yourself on the road while being far away in another decade.

Muscle memory makes up much of what we do. Unlike conscious memory, muscle memory is stored in a number of different areas of the brain, including the motor cortex, the basal ganglia, and the cerebellum. The system is separate and backed up in different ways. In other words, even if you lose all your conscious memories, you can still retain your muscle memories.[xciv]

So you want to maximize the muscle memory you have. It's a backup system for the conscious brain. I'm convinced that the reason older people don't like to travel and are happiest at home has to do with gradual dependence more and more on our muscle memories. I don't have to think about where something is in the house. I just need to let my body take me there. The laundry is done this way, because that's the way the door always opens. This faucet always sticks, while this one is loose. Every day there are ten thousand things that I rely on my muscle memory to help me process. Without that fall back, traveling in a strange place, I have to adjust, to process all this new information. Even if the trip is perfect, it's stressful. So many new faucets, so much new information about bedding, room location, and when is breakfast again?

But rather than feeling bad about muscle memory, we should exploit it to its fullest extent. Everything in its place. The previous owner of my house went so far as to build cabinets for specific tasks. I use the yarn cabinet for other things, but I appreciate the holes he drilled for his wife to help her keep the yarn sorted. One of the wisest things I ever did in my house is install hooks for every key. You see these at older hotels (where they still have real keys). But in my house the keys would wander all over the messy kitchen counter or even stay in coat pockets. Morning was a game of bad Easter Egg hunting with the prize being getting to work on time. Now I hang up my keys without thinking about it. It's automatic. It's a muscle memory.

How much of your life can be automated? Why not take a moment to figure out how to do something the best way, then agree on the way something will be done? After that, just do things in the same way. Before you know it, the tool got back to its niche, the dish towels are right where they're supposed to be, and the food that you needed got ordered. It all happened with the minimum of conscious effort.

Let's be clear, my goal is not for you to forget your life. It's to free up your life to remember the things you want to remember. Do you really need to spend thirty minutes hunting for the remote? Or should you attach velcro to the back and hang it on the chair where it gets used? No, it's not a perfect solution. It's just a better solution than wandering from room to room until you find the remote next to the bread or sitting in the refrigerator because you needed that hand for the relish.

Think of muscle memory as your first line of defense against younglings who want to convince you to live in a home. Remote in the fridge? Time for the talk. Remote velcroed to the chair? No need for the talk. Dad is just as forgetful, just more functional about how he's living. And being functional is the key to staying in your home. So automate everything you can.

MAXIMIZING YOUR SHORT-TERM MEMORY

OK, so you've removed the silly clutter from your short-term memory. Things are in their place, you aren't stressed, and you're ready to remember.

The process of remembering is the process of making connections. Literally in your brain, you want to connect different nerve cells. But that means you need to make conscious connections between what you want to remember and as many different areas of your brain as you can.

Let's pick something a little more useful to talk about. At 30 degrees Fahrenheit, with a wind of 30 miles an hour, the actual temperature is 15 degrees, and you'll get frostbite in 30 minutes. You've got a bit more time than that, but who wants to play around with frostbite?

When I think about these numbers, there's lots of thirties. I might just remember 30/30/30, and see my hands turning blue at 30 (sight). While I do that, I rub my hands together (touch). I say out loud "30/30/30, get inside" (hearing). Because I've got nothing else, I smell my hands, which smell like my conditioner, and rub them again (smell) while saying "30/30/30, get inside." I'm not going to make you lick your fingers (taste), because that's just weird, but it will probably help you remember to get inside when the wind is blowing hard below freezing.

Now, I can increase my memory of that fact by shifting it from declarative (facts) to episodic (emotions) by adding an emotion. I'll pick fear. So now I rub my hands together, picture them blue, blow on them, and say fearfully, "30/30/30, get inside!"

Good, now I've got a short term memory. It should last me for an hour or so, unless something stressful happens to wipe it out. If I want to remember it longer. I would refresh the memory in an hour, and again in another day. Come back to it every week for a couple of months and I've got a new permanent fixture in my mind. One of my early readers of this book said it sounds like her mother's instructions for maintaining a wooden butcher block. It should be oiled once a day for a week, once a week for a month, once a month for a year, and once a year for the rest of her life. I like the idea of "oiling" our memories regularly, keeping them working rather than expecting them to start up at a moment's notice after decades of neglect.

DEFAULT MODE NETWORK REWIRE

What about continuously trying to remember? Forcing myself to remember all day? Not as useful as you'd think. The brain doesn't work that way.

We think we're going to remember better the more active, the more aggressive we are. But we'll have to work twice as hard if we don't give our brains time away from the subject.

Why? The brain doesn't have downtime. When you give your brain downtime, your brain goes into something called the default mode networking state. That's when it processes everything you've done all day, and decides how it really sees that material. You need to be going into default mode daily to do things like confirm your own identity, understand other people's behavior, and create an internal code of ethics. Don't worry, your body uses sleep time to do most of this processing, but it will take any downtime you give it to do this work. Most creative people need breaks during the day to do precisely this kind of deeper work.[xcv] What's happening during daydreaming is the rerunning of the neural circuits in your head. The brain is making them more efficient, more effective. It's fine tuning your memories. Pushing yourself for more than an hour (expert level performers max out at about four hours of training a day) can result in burnout. In comparison, "the first night of sleep after learning has a particularly important effect on memory."[xcvi]

The most efficient way to try to remember something is to repeat it, check it again in twenty minutes, go over it in the evening, again the next day, and then repeat it once every few days after that. Once it's solid in the long-term memory, then simply attach a number of different ways of remembering it, different "doors" to access the same information. (Different senses, different associations with people, with locations, etc.) Once you've done that, you should have a brand new memory that will stay with you for some time.

SIMPLE REPETITION MADE EASY

Let's say you ignore everything else in this book, and you just want to make remembering things like test answers easier. Turns out, you're not the first person to want to do this particular feat of memory.

A gentleman named Hermann Ebbinghaus was the first person to have subjected someone to endless memorizing of nonsense words to see how fast the subject forgot the words. He can be forgiven, because he used himself as a subject. I can only imagine what it must have been like in his house with papa mumbling nonsense to himself. With that kind of upbringing, of course his son had to become a philosopher.[xcvii] But Ebbinghaus came up with the learning curve, which we still talk about today. He also came up with the forgetting curve, which we seem to have forgotten. One of the key things about Ebbinghaus' forgetting curve was that once he forgot all his nonsense words, relearning them was still much faster than starting from scratch. He proved that the material was still stored in his brain somewhere, he just couldn't access it. Ebbinghaus' flaw in his research was that he only had himself as a subject. But other researchers have repeated his experiments with similar results.[xcviii]

Since Ebbinghaus, other researchers have tightened the boundaries on maximum learning of things like dates and times of great cheese-based inventions. They have found that the optimal timing of reviewing material depends on how long you want to remember the material. If you need to remember things for a week, then looking at them again in a day or two is ideal. But if you want to remember things for a year, then reviewing the material a month later will be better. If you want to remember things for several years, then several months should go by before you review the material again. Anyone who remembers school will recall how short the period was between learning and testing. No wonder we're not producing students who retain the material from year to year. For those of us who are in charge of our own memories, coming back to material a few months later is both easier and more effective. One large study of memory found that waiting several months doubled the memory retention of subjects years later.[xcix]

HOW DO WE KEEP OUR MEMORIES?

The way we lose our memories can direct us to specific processes on how to retain them. Think back to how you lose your memories. The minor and unimportant goes away first. So concern and focus on retaining these memories should result in better retention. Techniques like visualizing people's names on their foreheads in flaming letters can help you remember their names. Adding an emotion to that memory can help you hold onto it more.

RAISING THE STAKES

The same things that make movies more entertaining also make your memories more memorable. Fred Burns is a boring name, but if Fred is literally burning, you'll remember his name in the elevator. Trying to remember a grocery list can seem impossible, but if it was attack of the mile high zucchini, you wouldn't forget to pick up a couple.

PRACTICE MEMORIZING ONE RIDICULOUS THING A DAY

Pick a fact, make it memorable by associating that fact with some crazy scene. It can be anything, but we tend to remember shocking sights more than simple ones. Something horrifying or disturbing like a sexy pink elephant will stay with you. (Now try not to think of the pink elephant. You can't, right? So apply the elephant to your grocery list.)

MEMORIZE THE NUMBERS TO LETTERS MEMORY SYSTEM (AND APPLY IT)

I read *The Memory Book* by Henry Lorayne and came away with this numbers to letters system that is at least several hundred years old. Lewis Carroll used another system, so I would pick one to memorize. Once you've made the association, you can use it to memorize numbers like your social security number or library card number. I used to practice on license plates to keep up my ability. The system is called the major system and in its most simple form associates the numbers like this: 0=S, 1=T/D, 2=N, 3=M, 4=R, 5=L, 6=SH/CH, 7=K, 8=F/PH, 9=P/B. The letters were chosen for common usage, but there is nothing magical about that particular association. You could use a musical scale or a set of pictures instead. I simply memorized the association. So something like 740184352 becomes KRSTFR MLN or Christopher Maloney. It takes some initial effort, but it trains the mind with a different pathway for remembering numbers in the short term memory, which is well worth knowing.

14 What Should We Take?

Now we really speculate.

Start with the facts. The big researchers say that, "We did not find evidence that any vitamin or mineral supplementation strategy for cognitively healthy adults in mid or late life has a meaningful effect on cognitive decline or dementia."[c]

So before you shell out for the newest squid spleen supplement that cures memory loss, let me sell you on this one. The supplement I'm thinking of has been used successfully without toxicity by millions of people. It has been shown to enhance cognitive functioning,[ci] reverses oxidative damage in the brain,[cii] and extracts of this supplement taken up the nose work as well as a drug for treating Alzheimer's disease.[ciii] The side effects include better nutrient absorption and better bowel function. When tested, it doesn't interact or conflict with common drugs,[civ] and may help them absorb better.[cv] Sound amazing?

Now available at the home shopping network: it's black pepper. So maybe the nurse in Alice In Wonderland knew what she was doing when she kept adding more pepper to the soup.

The information on pepper and dementia is extensive. It combines and supports the function of both turmeric[cvi] and quercetin, which are also possibly helpful treatments. Quercetin combined with pepper reversed brain damage in rats.[cvii]

We don't have large human trials on pepper, but we do have

dog trials. The dogs were either left in a control group or fed turmeric, green tea, NAC, alpha-lipoic acid, and black pepper. After three months, the older dogs on the supplement showed a significantly higher attention span and showed fewer errors on testing.[cviii] When the researchers paired the old dogs against young dogs, it turns out that it does take longer to teach an old dog new tricks. But adding the supplement did help them remember better.[cix]

Given the possible benefit of statin drugs for memory, a person might reasonably assume that inflammation of the brain causes much of the problem. Small studies show that inflammation markers are higher in people with dementia (but not AD).[cx] But other small studies show that the things we'd take for inflammation don't help. Aspirin didn't help and caused more bleeding. NSAIDS (Tylenol, Advil, etc.) caused a host of problems without helping. And Cox-2 Inhibitors made things worse than NSAIDS.[cxi] So there is inflammation, but it's not inflammation that can be treated well with a drug.

Supplements have been tried for dementia, including "antioxidants, B-vitamins, inositol, medium-chain triglyceride, omega-3, polymeric formulas, polypeptides, and vitamin D." The polypeptides and the B-vitamins did seem to help a bit, but not enough to really credit them with much benefit. At the same time, insufficient levels of vitamins, like vitamin D, can make dementia worse.[cxii] As with all vitamins, if you're deficient, correcting the deficiency can be a miracle. If you're not, your body is likely just going to process them through. Dementia is not a vitamin deficiency except in very rare cases.[cxiii]

When we don't have good options in Western medicine, it can be tempting to look to Chinese medicine or other alternatives. Herbs like Ginkgo biloba, Huperzine A (Lycopodium serratum) and Ginseng show promise for dementia. But the benefits have not been shown to be consistent, so it's hard to know how much benefit to expect.[cxiv] The herbs are often promoted for their similarity to existing drugs, like how an extract of daffodil bulbs (Galantamine, marketed as Reminyl) has similar effects to donepezil, rivastigmine, and tacrine. These are all cholinesterase inhibitors, it's just that the first one was originally naturally derived. So they all have similar effects and side effects.[cxv] And the drugs' effects are "not clinically meaningful."[cxvi] The daffodil bulb extract has been associated with a possible increased death rate.[cxvii]

Let's take a moment to go over the supplements Dr. Bredesen gives to his patients as part of his cure. Not because you should take them, but because it's good to know what all your friends will be horking down every morning in an effort to keep their memories. Remember, these are the supplements that are included in his *The End of Alzheimer's* book, so we're picking the best of the best.

Dr. Bredesen has a large number of supplements: coconut oil, resveratrol, B vitamins, Selenium, CoQ10, vitamin C, Omega 3s, Vitamin E, Vitamin D, and NAC. He also adds in a number of herbs: Gotu kolu, turmeric, Ashwaghanda, and Lion's Mane mushroom.

Coconut oil for memory? In 2017, a small single blind study says it helps a bit.[cxviii] Another small study found it helped women with moderate dementia?[cxix] Maybe in place of olive oil in a Mediterranean diet?

How about resveratrol? There's a lot of discussion of what it should be able to do for dementia, but no human studies. The small studies we do have cover resveratrol as part of a French diet, including nuts, vegetables, oranges, berries, soy, and olive oil. That diet seemed to help with dementia.[cxx]

B vitamins for dementia? If you're deficient (have abnormal blood) yes, they're helpful. They might be helpful otherwise, but the researchers weren't convinced. They did say that B vitamins were better with omega 3s added, and that of all the supplements researched in the last ten years only B vitamins showed benefit.[cxxi] What are good sources of B vitamins? Meats, seeds and nuts, whole grains, dark leafy green vegetables, and fruits.

What about selenium for memory? We have negative evidence here, with a recent check of people with dementia showing no relation to selenium levels at all.[cxxii] Another study found dumping people with dementia full of selenium might have slowed decline, but they weren't sure.[cxxiii] These results are disappointing given earlier good results with mice. So if you pet mouse has dementia, selenium might be a good option. Just not for grandma. If you must, fish and nuts are good sources of selenium.

CoQ10 has such a sexy reputation. How does it do for memory? Not a good treatment, because dementia patients don't show a deficiency. Might be a predictor of higher risk (because of the connection to heart disease).[cxxiv] Good sources of CoQ10 are meats, vegetables, fruits, and beans.

Vitamin C has almost magical powers. Does it reverse memory loss? Patients with dementia were low in vitamin E, not in vitamin C or vitamin A.[cxxv] Researchers looking at fifty studies found slightly higher vitamin C levels in people without dementia, but there was no connection between vitamin C levels and dementia itself.[cxxvi] The best source of vitamin C is citrus fruit, which is 95% absorbed (compared to 5-10% absorption from a supplement).

Omega 3 fatty acids are critical for the brain, right? I have to admit I was hopeful for this supplement, and there's roughly five times the amount of research on this treatment and dementia. But the big reviews are not positive. They talk about a "lack of convincing evidence" in all the big trials.[cxxvii] Another review found maybe a benefit for people just starting with dementia, which sounds like someone trying to make things look better than they are.[cxxviii] But all the research is based on the observation than people who eat more fish have less dementia.[cxxix] So maybe we should be eating the fish, not the pills?

OK, vitamin E is lower in dementia patients. So does supplementing with vitamin E help them? We've known about the connection for fifty years, but we don't have any evidence that more E slows dementia.[cxxx] It might help with functional living for people with advanced dementia, and its side effect picture is similar to placebo.[cxxxi] So this is one that I might give to someone far advanced?

Vitamin D is a big player these days in the vitamin world. Does it help with memory? Even in patients with low vitamin D levels, supplementing with vitamin D over six months did not help with memory.[cxxxii] Another study tracking people over twenty years found that lower vitamin D did not result in more dementia.[cxxxiii]

How about NAC? I think of it as more of a help cleaning up the brain, but maybe that's what the brain needs to help with memory. There's a lot of medical chatter about the potential of NAC to help with a lot of brain problems, including dementia, and the wording of the different abstracts is suspiciously similar. I'm not saying that some manufacturer is paying to have NAC positively reviewed, just that I'm concerned. There may be a new drug in the pipeline that uses NAC as a base.[cxxxiv] As far as dementia is concerned, there may be some positive rat studies, but nothing for humans yet.[cxxxv] Foods high in NAC like compounds are broccoli, asparagus and most high protein foods.

Well, that's Dr. Bredesen's list. If you noticed a theme, it should be: eat food not supplements. I really, really wish he'd focused people on making the dietary changes rather than pushing the supplements, because there isn't strong support for anything he's recommending.

Simple answer on supplements: eat Mediterranean, check with your doctor for deficiencies. Otherwise, don't worry about it.

15 My Plan For Memory

So what am I going to do to keep my memory? Funny thing, I'm going to do more funny things. What I've learned says that crosslinking our memories to multiple pathways means better retention but -more importantly- more ready access. If you can access that memory from three or four directions, it's much better as a memory. Single directional memories do very little to help us remember. One lost connection, and you might as well not have done it at all.

So the key is not to try and learn things in a vacuum. We need to learn things in context, with our senses. That means experiencing the world, not watching it on a screen. Learn your facts while out in nature, engage your mind and your body in every learning task. When you want to remember something, you want your brain to light up like a symphony, not have one red dot where that memory is stored. It's not just use it or lose it, it's strengthen it and diversify it.

MOVEMENT BEATS MEMORIZATION

Let's say we want to memorize a list of animals. We could sit down and start reading the list. Then we can say the list out loud to ourselves. We can add emotion to our voices, and eventually we'll have a memorized list.

But what if instead we act out the list. Cat, dog, rooster, cow. Remember that ancient spinning toy that went around and made those sounds? If you do, first you're as old as the hills like me. And two, if you think back all the animals I just mentioned are on that toy. The reason I can remember them decades later is because of the spinning. Over the years I've had to bark like a dog or moo like a cow dozens of other times (as anyone who has had kids will attest). But I never had to spin over and over to get the sound I wanted. The repetition of movement cemented that toy, those sounds, and that list of animals in my brain. Goat, bird, sheep, what else made up that loop? Nope, no goat. Frog, coyote, horse, duck, pig, and turkey all had their sounds. They have a newer version with things like alligator, which I think makes a hissing sound like a snake? The point is that old people wander, but that these long term memories tied to movement stay with us after decades. So act out the things you want to remember. If you're trying to recall something, particularly something you've set down, go back to the original door you came in. Act as if you have the thing in your hand, and walk into the room again. Look around to where you would have set it down. The likeliest solution is that it's still there, or slightly covered by some other object so that it's not readily visible.

MUSIC

I have been blessed by children who have required of me the simplest and most memorable of memory exercises: an instrument.

My older son took up the violin. I, who had only a single lesson in violin when I was in elementary school, was helpless to help him. So I purchased a cheap violin and began lessons along with him. We even performed once together and the listeners commented that I made more mistakes than he did (I didn't tell them I'd started at the same time).

After years and many sizes of violins, I was excited to start my younger son. I thought I'd finally be ahead of the learning curve. But he didn't like the violin, and wanted a cello. So I've learned the cello for the last six years.

Learning a musical instrument as an adult is a lesson in humility and humiliation. Older fingers and older brains are not as nimble. My son can memorize a song in a tenth of the time. He actually improves when he hasn't been playing. I only get worse the longer I'm away from the instrument.

But I know that the learning affects my brain. It literally makes my head tired, an impossibility since the brain has no sensory nerves. But it does. I need a break after a strenuous effort, and I've seen both my sons need a similar break. Music is to the brain what weights are for the arms.

MEMORY LANE

What I've learned is that scrapbooks aren't optional. My wife has collected a series of photo albums, overpriced wastes of time that I now cherish. Rather than ignore them, I'm going to pick one up, a different one every month, and go through it with her. I'll add notes, strengthen connections, and build the web of memory in my mind. My life is as important to me as any test, and I now know that the things we want to remember we need to practice remembering.

DIET AND LIFESTYLE

For many of you, converting to a Mediterranean diet may be a struggle. I've been there for years. So as part of that journey I'm going to work on creating a cookbook for all of you, so you can not only follow the basics you can also see what sort of crazy food I eat. If at any point you need to stop sugar or gluten or decide that all God's creatures are family, you'll be prepared.

I also exercise regularly, but I'm going to increase my memory walks. Currently I'll go around my neighborhood and be off in my head. But now I'm going to walk around remembering. Looking at the place where we had the sled accident, where my son took his senior photos, where we had the outdoor birthday party. Instead of escaping my surroundings, I'm going to marinate in them. Soak in the memories, make the ties all over again. Like an old knit sweater, I'm going to repair any minor tears before they get bigger.

What I'm not going to do is take a lot of supplements. The one

I'm considering is bringing back in vitamin B12. It along with vitamin D are the things I get short of as a vegan in a Maine winter. I expect I'll take them for a while to see if they affect how I feel, then taper off them and see if I feel any worse. It's this model of supplement taking, the "I notice a difference" model, that I most respect. It bypasses all the "it should do this or that" hoopla and cuts right to the individual's personal response.

MEMORY GAMES
INCREASING BRAIN SPEED

The first thing I did when I wanted to improve my own memory was to look up memory speed training. Why? Because it can save your life. If we believe a three year study on memory speed training, one five week course has results that last up to three years. I defy any muscle exercise routine anywhere on the internet to give you those kinds of results. But that wasn't the reason I went looking for speed training first. Patients who did the five week course had an impressive 40% reduction in car accidents. Not bad for a two hours a week for five weeks, then nothing more.[cxxxvi]

You'd think a game that successful would be easy to find, but you'd be wrong. The research articles themselves don't list the games, so you have to go searching.

If you look up memory speed training online you don't find brain speed, you find computer speed. But the definition is relevant. The faster the processing speed, the faster your computer (or your brain) can react to orders.

Add a specific search for brain speed, and what we find are studies on whether or not playing with your phone while walking affects memory. It turns out young healthy volunteers aren't terribly troubled memory wise by walking and texting.[cxxxvii] The researchers didn't test how these same volunteers would fare if they were wandering in traffic.

You can also find reports that brain exercises don't work...for young healthy volunteers. Or more precisely, they don't work generally if you do specific exercises.[cxxxviii] Getting faster at recognizing a red light doesn't raise your IQ. Anyone who thought his IQ would go up from playing video games might want to avoid buying a bridge in Brooklyn. But getting faster at recognizing a red light...makes you faster at recognizing a red light. And that can be lifesaving if you need to get faster at seeing a red light.

Eventually I tracked down the original video game. It's called Road Tour and is sold by Posit Games. Posit Games is now BrainHQ,[cxxxix] and they have a range of exercises. I gave them my email, and they let me do a free speed training exercise. It flashed a dark bird with a bunch of light birds faster and faster until it was almost impossible to see it. But I got five stars, and I assume every day I will get a new free exercise of the day. I do, with daily reminders to sign up. But the first two days are the same exercise, and by the third day the exercise didn't work. The fourth day gave me the same exercise of spotting birds so quickly they can barely register, so they're clearly not rotating through all the exercises available. I've seen this with many programs, where they have freebies that don't function, but it doesn't speak well of the entire program. The program also has monthly subscriptions, which seem reasonable. So a purist would say do the exact thing that the study did (one hour twice a week) and nothing else.

In comparison, another online company, Cognifit, offered me a free twenty minute memory test. My scores put me at older than my age. But let's look at those scores together.

"Attention 448/800 Perception 392/800 Reasoning 335/800
Memory 241/800 Coordination 187/800"

Do you see my worst score? Coordination. I wasn't fast with my mouse. Given that all of these tests are based on timed mouse clicks and I was accurate in remembering up to seven numbers, I'm not sure how to judge their results other than to get a better mouse. Basically, they're testing mouse-click speed over and over again. I can't imagine how well I'd do on my "memory training" after an hour of rapid mouse clicking. The poor computer would be flashing up ads for assisted care and Alzheimer's specialists. But somehow I don't think my best memory booster lifestyle change would be to get a better mouse.

It's still interesting to see how you did on different tests, and the free Cognifit trial make me look at things differently. It starts me thinking about how I think. Some of my scores were decent, while others needed a lot of work. My strengths included things I've been practicing on other programs over the last few days, "Divided

Attention 800, Spatial Perception 702, and Visual Perception 582." My weaknesses included "Visual Short Term Memory 67, Short-Term Memory 169, and Processing Speed 172." So that's good information to go looking for other memory programs that might address my worst scores. Or is it? I just went to the most difficult short-term memory game and cleared it in under six minutes.[cxl] So I have to think that all Cognifit tests is my mouse hand speed, which is very disturbing for a group that claims they're helping people with memory. I imagine a patient who can't feed herself but who has a quick mouse hand might get a good score on their test. And yes, I expect in a couple of days I will become much better at any of these games. I'll probably go back in a month and see how I did, without signing up for the program.

These websites want me to commit for a month or even a year at a time. Personally, that's not going to work for me. I know from my own history online that I tend to binge on these things and be very motivated for about two weeks. Then I forget to do the games going forward. So for now I'm either going to do one exercise a day or nothing at all. But if I was having trouble, I'd be on that site or one of its competitors for the prescribed five weeks. There are many, and most of them seem to follow the same style of common exercises "proven" to be best for an aging brain. When I did something like test for my brain age, I found that some exercises are much more difficult for me than others.[cxli] I also found that even the second time through I was faster. My brain was smarter about how it played, and I learned tricks to exploit weaknesses in the game.

The difficulty with the memory exercises for adults is that they're...well...boring. They're good for you, like bran cereal. But I'm not going to get excited about recognizing a dark bird. My brain will be tired after an hour, but I'm not going to think, "Oh boy, I get to try and recognize the dark bird faster tomorrow."

Now, researchers analyzing all the brain training studies found that most of the brain training games online overhype their benefit, particularly for young, healthy adults. To quote one researcher, Elizabeth Stine-Morrow, "Does brain training work? Yes, it's called school."[cxlii]

Yep, there's a group of people that we actively make do brain exercises every day. They just happen to be between five and twenty-five. If you go online to search for memory games for children, there are all sorts of free online games. One site of many I found had games like Simon (recognizing green and red lights at increasing speed) and an eyesight challenge, where you try and spot your keys or other objects in a cluttered room. I also liked the jumping arrows challenge, where they switch the directions of the arrows on you so that you have to recognize the change at faster and faster speeds.[cxliii] There are also dozens of driving games, including first person games where you're driving down the highway at a hundred miles an hour and avoiding crashing. Put something like that on a Wii with a driving wheel, and I'm having a hard time seeing how that wouldn't be helpful on your driving response times.

Researchers point out that solitary online games lack the context of a classroom, where brain stimulation takes place on multiple levels. The same researchers singled out the ACTIVE study (which forms the basis of many of this book's recommendations) for its high quality. It showed improvement for older adults in the areas they trained in over an extended period of time. While the researchers would have liked every study to meet the same standard, the ACTIVE study cost millions of dollars and lasted a decade. It's unlikely any online gaming company could invest that kind of money into research and development. But we don't need them to, we just need to have them drop the hype and focus on what they're really training the brain to do. To quote the highly critical review of all brain studies, "(W)e find extensive evidence that brain-training interventions improve performance on the trained tasks."[cxliv] It was the broader application of that training that they didn't agree was happening. Just as learning to row a boat won't necessarily help you learn to dance, speed recognition training won't necessarily help you learn Swahili. That's reasonable, and we shouldn't expect that kind of crossover effect. The fact that speed training over the next five weeks could affect how you drive in two years is in itself pretty impressive. (A critical review pointed out that this benefit only resulted in a few less accidents, but did not question the overall results.)

Since few speed training exercises will have the same backing as the ACTIVE trial, it makes sense to question any new online exercise. Critics are right that social context, spending time with friends, and going back to school are superior to doing something online for your brain. But whether doing something or nothing is better is also clear. In a small study, researchers tested both a brain game and a placebo brain game. Both the gamers and the placebo gamers improved in a similar way. In other words, there is no placebo. Doing something with your brain will improve your brain.[cxlv] Engaging your brain is always going to be a better choice than doing nothing.

OK, we can see short-term results and even some moderate longer effects, but do we have evidence that brain training can change the brain's structure? Yes. Researchers look for changes in the hippocampus, a seahorse-shaped area at the base of the brain that is most dramatically impacted by Alzheimer's disease. To do this, they had seniors with early dementia participate in three hours a week of a multicomponent exercise program. Seniors learned a range of new tasks in combination with age appropriate aerobic exercise (treadmill, senior volleyball, dancing). At the end of six months, the participants had a 10% increase in brain thickness and better blood flow. The control group lost 2% of their brain function in the same period.[cxlvi] Maybe we should change "use it or lose it" to "make it stronger and live longer."

16 Where Do We Go From Here?

There won't be a medical cure for dementia as long as we remain fixated on the damage in the brain as causing memory loss rather than being just a symptom of that loss.

The technophiles among us might dream of a day when we insert ourselves into computer memory banks and live our lives in an eternal state of mental clarity. I shared that dream until I read an article on just how complex our brains are. Remember when I said that computers are like a big room with lots of lights with on/off switches. The brain is like a much bigger room with all the lights on dimmer switches?

Just this year a group created a fake human brain with one hundred million switches. It's really impressive, took twenty years to build, and cost about fifteen million dollars. But it's not really a human brain. The supercomputer has roughly the same number of switches as a mouse.[cxlvii] A human brain is a thousand times more complex. So in order to create a human brain computer to receive the thoughts and memories of a single human is going to be far more expensive and complicated. We're going to need to completely rethink how we make supercomputers to even come close (hint: use a dimmer switch model, not on/off, computer guys).

In the meantime, we're on our own. Medicine will be wringing its hands and be buried under a deluge of dementia. (Stock picks for the future: nursing homes.) Technology is light years from being able to save us from ourselves.

I think at this point it might be wise to tell a story about E.B. White. His name came up as one of the famous people who suffered from Alzheimer's disease. Unlike the other famous people, I've felt a connection to E.B. White my whole life. He was part of *Shrunk and White's Elements of Style*, a pithy little grammar book worthy of rereading. While White is most famous for Charlotte's Web, I've always admired his Stuart Little, about the plucky mouse who inexplicably is born to human parents. White also lived in Maine, where I now reside. He's also a far better author than I am.

But E.B. White died of Alzheimer's disease, an odd thing for a person dedicated to letters. How could someone who used it all his life lose it at the end?

The answer in his case was a bump on the head. A blow from a canoe while he was loading it. The blow sent him reeling and made him confused. He never fully recovered, and his family never pursued further testing.

E.B. White himself did not pursue further testing because he was depressed. His wife Katharine had died several years earlier, and E.B. felt alone despite being surrounded by extended family. "I don't have friends here my own age. Everybody I know is below ground."[cxlviii]

One of E.B. White's sons disputes the Alzheimer's diagnosis. "(H)e took to his bed and never again knew exactly where he was. It looked like a rapid onset of Alzheimer's, but more likely, the doctors thought, was a senile dementia brought on by the blow to his head that day….died the next October, still at home and able to recognize the people around him....he enjoyed listening to his own writings, though he wasn't always clear about who the author was."[cxlix]

We should all be so fortunate, to pass away at home surrounded by loved ones, and still able to recognize them. But what is clear from this story is that E.B. White did not pass from dementia alone. Another man who had a wife who was still living might have gone to Boston to pursue more testing. The unspoken agreement was that it was time for E.B. White to go. He wasn't happy, he didn't want to stay. His life had ended with the loss of his lifelong love, and he was living on borrowed time.

My young son asked me about memory loss, and I told him that memory loss occurs after decades of not using your mind. Not months, not even a few years. Dementia comes on after decades of slow deterioration, sometimes visible to the doctors, sometimes invisible. There are those who resist it until they die of other causes. But it is a subtle and continuous loss, like a slow drip, that affects us all as we let go of our lives.

Yes, there are other causes of dementia. The early onset, rapid course of Alzheimer's is not memory loss. It is an organic attack on the brain from outside forces.

But the standard memory loss of age-related dementia is a loss that is predictable. In some ways it is a loss that is a blessing. We forget our lives before we leave them, a fuzzy blanket of confusion that relieves us of the need to stay, to live through the constant companion pains of old age. If we recognize that memory loss happens decades before the brain responds, then the holes and scarring of the brain are just the outer manifestations of an internal process well underway.

So we'll keep our memories if we care enough to try. What about the population as a whole? As we triple the number of people with dementia, there will no longer be wards and closed rooms for them.

Imagine a town square. It reminds you of the 1950's, a beautiful movie set. The people who live in this town are slower than you'd think, and need to be cared for more by others. But compared to any current medical model, they are less medicated, more joyful, eat better, and live longer.

Welcome to the future, to towns where people with dementia can live safely without fear. The prototype already exists, a place called Hogewey in the Netherlands. Patients can go to the post office, attend the theater, or visit with friends at a restaurant. All protected and cared for around the clock.[cl] That's how dementia ends, with all of the patients in *The Truman Show*, playing out a version of *50 First Dates* for the rest of their lives.

As we close, I want to leave you with a sense that things can turn around, not just for us individually, but for the world as a whole.

A recent major study of dementia progression found that recent dementia rates in the U.S. were dropping, not rising. Instead of the expected 11 percent rate, the rate was only 9 percent. So were people doing the "full Bredesen" or something similar?

No.

Were we healthier overall?

No.

We were worse. "23% of US adults were obese in 1990 compared with 35% in 2012; among adults 65 years or older, the prevalence of diabetes increased from 9% to 21%."[cli]

So we were sicker, older, fatter, in worse shape in every way, but our dementia rates dropped.

It's not just the one study. A follow up of the Framingham study found the rates of dementia have been dropping over the last thirty years. It's not because New Englanders got healthier. They were older and sicker, but had less dementia. The researchers can only shrug.[clii]

The simplest answer is that older people are staying sharper because they're trying to stay sharper. All this new technology is forcing new learning. Just managing a smartphone would have flummoxed one of our ancestors. But we expect grandma to not only call, she's also got to text and video chat.

I'd like to think that older people are also taking the time to work against memory loss, actively trying to use it so they won't lose it. But I suspect the necessity of modern living is forcing our brains to be stronger and so they're lasting longer.

Thanks for reading!

Appendix A: What Is Alzheimer's?

I wanted to know what Alzheimer's disease really was. The disease was named for Alois Alzheimer, who gave a lecture on a patient in 1906. In the lecture Alzheimer talked about a woman who had died young of dementia. Her brain showed thinning, senile plaques, and neurofibrillary tangles much more common in older dementia patients. These brain markers became the clear signs of Alzheimer's disease. They continued to be the standard markers of Alzheimer's disease right up to the year 2011.[cliii]

In 2011, the definition of Alzheimer's disease fundamentally changed. Even in 1984, experts had defined the disease based on Alois Alzheimer's plaques and tangles. They expected dead patients with worse dementia to show more plaques and more tangles. But it was clear that "Extensive AD pathology, particularly diffuse amyloid plaques, can be present in the absence of any obvious symptoms."[cliv] In other words, Alois Alzheimer was wrong in thinking that the plaques caused the dementia. They don't. But that throws out a hundred years of research, so the experts are redefining Alzheimer's disease to match what they currently know.

One of the most important changes made in 2011 was the recognition that memory loss occurs well before positive brain scans and that most other dementias do not look like Alzheimer's disease. Alzheimer's disease itself commonly coexists with blood vessel and Lewy body dementias, which led to the previous confusion about symptoms overlapping.

The amyloid plaque connection that Alzheimer noted has no connection to memory loss, and the neurofibrillary tangles are a better judge of how bad things are. But a better marker is synapse loss, the loss of connections between cells of the brain. Around 30% of normal memory older adults show all the pathological changes of Alzheimer's disease. On scans they show up with "amyloid positivity" despite no signs of memory loss. Experts still point out that around 30% of older adults also show up with dementia a decade later, but that connection literally places the cart before the horse. It says that the brain scans eventually "catch up to you" without any evidence that this is the case.

To maintain the connection to plaques, the experts now offer a convoluted explanation. Plaques can show up ten to twenty years before memory loss, while tangles and tau markers show up later on. The combination of the three getting progressively worse indicates a worsening of the brain damage.

If you notice, the experts have said there is no connection to plaques, then reinstated that connection to plaques as memory loss progresses. It shows how pervasive the Alzheimer model has become even after it's been disproven.[clv] To quote the experts, "Although it is possible that β-amyloid plaques and neurofibrillary tau deposits are not causal in AD pathogenesis, it is these abnormal protein deposits that define AD as a unique neurodegenerative disease."[clvi]

In 2018, expert researchers recommended defining Alzheimer's disease entirely by these biomarkers without any connection to clinical symptoms or memory loss. It frees up research into possible causes, but also divorces Alzheimer's research from any need to affect memory loss.

The critics of this new direction point out the disturbing lack of relevance in a commentary, "When Is Alzheimer's Not Dementia?" What it means for patients is that Alzheimer's research will progress into the theoretical rather than the curative, allowing researchers to keep researching plaques despite no connection to memory loss.[clvii] The argument for this approach is that it could be worthwhile; the argument against it is that we don't have time for researchers to explore every medical dead end. It's time to move on from Alois Alzheimer's 1906 observations and recognize that he was wrong about cause and effect in dementia.

LATE ONSET VS. EARLY ONSET ALZHEIMER'S DISEASE

Since 1937, we've known that the major signs for dementia in older patients are depression and memory loss. Late onset Alzheimer's disease happens after 65, and will eventually affect one in three older adults. Of those late onsetters, 98% are clinically depressed as well as suffering from memory loss.[clviii] They show up with those symptoms more than a decade before they show any signs of Alzheimer's disease, which we now know can take another ten years to really affect the memory. Taking a step back, we're talking about people who show up with depression after 65 and may have twenty years of severe depression and gradual memory loss before they are clinically diagnosed with Alzheimer's disease. The "will to live," while not a clinical term, comes to mind with these patients. Two decades of lacking significant social connections or any life purpose will severely affect even a twenty-year-old.

In comparison, early onset Alzheimer's disease affects less than 5% of patients, has a much higher genetic connection, and the patients are rarely depressed (8%) while suffering memory loss. But arguing that even early onset Alzheimer's is largely genetic doesn't hold water. There are clinical cases of identical twins, one of whom dies of early onset Alzheimer's and the other one who remains normal.[clix]

There is a rare, rapidly progressive form of Alzheimer's disease that was previously misdiagnosed as Creutzfeldt-Jakob disease (CJD). It includes muscle jerking, muscle spasms, and rapid changes in how a person walks. From my own research, I am suspicious about this illness being more infectious in nature.[clx]

But we shouldn't waste our time worrying about extremely rare disease possibilities when we have a clear framework for how we can keep our memories.

Thanks for reading!

ABOUT THE AUTHOR

Dr. Christopher Maloney, N.D., saw patients in family practice in Portland and Augusta Maine before finding out he had colon cancer. Since his diagnosis he's dedicated himself to spending time with his family (and the occasional patient). He also changed his diet, exercises daily, and doesn't feel deprived. He hopes that each person reading his books will be helped.

He can be reached at docmaloneynd@gmail.com.
Nope, he cannot diagnose or treat your disease via the internet.
But he has hundreds of answers to common health questions at Alternative Holistic Health Answers, as well as answers on Quora.

If you enjoyed this book, please review it online.

Dr. Maloney has other books for the more general public that you can find anywhere electronic books are sold. Look for Christopher Maloney, CJ Maloney, and Roy LeRoy.

Thanks for reading!

The endnotes are in medline format rather than standard bibliographic format because I didn't want to double the size of this book with citations. Searching for pubmed with the identifying number will give you the original study abstract or the full paper.

[i] https://www.ncbi.nlm.nih.gov/pubmed/27840472

[ii] https://www.ncbi.nlm.nih.gov/pmc/articles/PMC5427593/

[iii] https://www.ncbi.nlm.nih.gov/pmc/articles/PMC2981103/

[iv] https://www.ncbi.nlm.nih.gov/pmc/articles/PMC3181710/

[v] https://www.ncbi.nlm.nih.gov/pmc/articles/PMC5946098/

[vi] https://content.iospress.com/articles/journal-of-alzheimers-disease/jad00175

[vii] https://www.ncbi.nlm.nih.gov/pubmed/26402763

[viii] https://www.mayoclinic.org/diseases-conditions/alzheimers-disease/in-depth/alzheimers-genes/art-20046552

[ix] https://www.ncbi.nlm.nih.gov/pubmed/30282369

[x] https://www.ncbi.nlm.nih.gov/pubmed/30530186

[xi] https://www.ncbi.nlm.nih.gov/pubmed/24634832

[xii] https://www.ncbi.nlm.nih.gov/pubmed/21284913

[xiii] https://dian.wustl.edu/our-research/observational-study/

[xiv] https://dian.wustl.edu/about/

[xv] https://www.bmj.com/content/340/bmj.c1425

[xvi] https://academic.oup.com/bmb/article/112/1/71/2747689

[xvii] https://academic.oup.com/psychsocgerontology/article/56/3/P141/2965072

[xviii] http://www.slate.com/articles/health_and_science/family/2014/03/dem

entia_and_aging_diary_of_a_sufferer_of_microvascular_disease.html

[xix] https://www.uml.edu/docs/Mini%20Mental%20State%20Exam_tcm18-169319.pdf

[xx] https://www.medpagetoday.com/neurology/dementia/52040

[xxi] https://academic.oup.com/jpubhealth/article/37/4/597/2362594

[xxii] https://www.ncbi.nlm.nih.gov/pubmed/20368517

[xxiii] https://academic.oup.com/bmb/article/112/1/71/2747689

[xxiv] https://www.ncbi.nlm.nih.gov/pubmed/24354019

[xxv] https://www.ncbi.nlm.nih.gov/pubmed/2943887

[xxvi] https://www.ncbi.nlm.nih.gov/pubmed/1479321

[xxvii] https://pdfs.semanticscholar.org/0fbd/039355147ebec2772de0fb512b b9b3573bfe.pdf

[xxviii] https://www.ncbi.nlm.nih.gov/pmc/articles/PMC2813509/

[xxix] https://www.ncbi.nlm.nih.gov/pubmed/28328043

[xxx] https://www.ncbi.nlm.nih.gov/pubmed/28328043

[xxxi] https://www.ncbi.nlm.nih.gov/pubmed/24354019

[xxxii] https://www.ncbi.nlm.nih.gov/pubmed/26091818

[xxxiii] https://www.ncbi.nlm.nih.gov/pubmed/25933023

[xxxiv] https://www.ncbi.nlm.nih.gov/pubmed/29131306

[xxxv] https://www.ncbi.nlm.nih.gov/pubmed/12391943

[xxxvi] http://english.prescrire.org/en/81/168/55126/0/NewsDetails.aspx

[xxxvii] https://www.ncbi.nlm.nih.gov/pubmed/30591071

[xxxviii] https://www.ncbi.nlm.nih.gov/pubmed/28527206

xxxix https://www.ncbi.nlm.nih.gov/pubmed/24354019

xl https://www.ncbi.nlm.nih.gov/pubmed/24531163

xli http://www.human-memory.net/types_sensory.html

xlii https://www.wired.com/2009/03/ff-perfectmemory/

xliii https://www.ncbi.nlm.nih.gov/pubmed/29125484

xliv https://www.ncbi.nlm.nih.gov/pubmed/29249209

xlv https://www.ncbi.nlm.nih.gov/pmc/articles/PMC6061119/

xlvi https://www.ncbi.nlm.nih.gov/pubmed/30025849

xlvii https://www.ncbi.nlm.nih.gov/pmc/articles/PMC6061119/

xlviii https://www.ncbi.nlm.nih.gov/pubmed/26294005

xlix https://www.ncbi.nlm.nih.gov/pmc/articles/PMC3857242/

l https://www.ncbi.nlm.nih.gov/pubmed/23924584

li https://www.ncbi.nlm.nih.gov/pubmed/29282641

lii https://www.ncbi.nlm.nih.gov/pubmed/29110906

liii https://www.ncbi.nlm.nih.gov/pubmed/19818896

liv https://www.ninds.nih.gov/Disorders/Patient-Caregiver-Education/Life-and-Death-Neuron

lv https://www.ncbi.nlm.nih.gov/pubmed/29869337

lvi https://www.ncbi.nlm.nih.gov/pubmed/18378330

lvii https://www.popularmechanics.com/science/health/a13017/how-much-of-the-brain-can-a-person-do-without-17223085/

lviii http://edition.cnn.com/2009/HEALTH/10/12/woman.brain/index.html?iref=24hours

lix http://newsroom.ucla.edu/releases/brain-re-wires-itself-after-damage-246049

lx http://drjilltaylor.com/book.html

lxi https://www.ted.com/talks/jill_bolte_taylor_s_powerful_stroke_of_insight?

lxii https://aging.ufl.edu/files/2011/01/deconditioning_campbell.pdf

lxiii https://www.ncbi.nlm.nih.gov/pmc/articles/PMC3268521/

lxiv https://www.nzherald.co.nz/lifestyle/news/article.cfm?c_id=6&objectid=11411570

lxv http://newsroom.ucla.edu/releases/memory-loss-associated-with-alzheimers-reversed-for-first-time

lxvi https://www.ncbi.nlm.nih.gov/pmc/articles/PMC4221920/

lxvii https://www.ncbi.nlm.nih.gov/pmc/articles/PMC3779441/

lxviii https://www.youtube.com/watch?v=6D5aA_-3Ip8 (minute 59)

lxix https://www.ncbi.nlm.nih.gov/pmc/articles/PMC4789584/

lxx https://www.ncbi.nlm.nih.gov/pmc/articles/PMC4586104/

lxxi https://www.ncbi.nlm.nih.gov/pubmed/30283265

lxxii http://newsroom.ucla.edu/releases/memory-loss-associated-with-alzheimers-reversed-for-first-time

lxxiii https://www.omicsonline.org/open-access/reversal-of-cognitive-decline-100-patients-2161-0460-1000450.pdf

lxxiv https://www.ncbi.nlm.nih.gov/pmc/articles/PMC1513668/

lxxv https://www.ornish.com/wp-content/uploads/Highmark-cost-analysis-2.pdf

lxxvi https://www.ncbi.nlm.nih.gov/pmc/articles/PMC4260956/

lxxvii https://www.ncbi.nlm.nih.gov/pmc/articles/PMC4888427/

lxxviii https://www.ncbi.nlm.nih.gov/pubmed/27031490

lxxix https://www.ncbi.nlm.nih.gov/pubmed/27236155

lxxx https://www.ncbi.nlm.nih.gov/pubmed/25961184

lxxxi https://www.ncbi.nlm.nih.gov/pubmed/23732551

lxxxii https://www.ncbi.nlm.nih.gov/pubmed/30181165

lxxxiii https://www.ncbi.nlm.nih.gov/pubmed/30497964

lxxxiv https://www.ncbi.nlm.nih.gov/pubmed/30094113

lxxxv https://www.ncbi.nlm.nih.gov/pubmed/8327020

lxxxvi https://www.ncbi.nlm.nih.gov/pubmed/12868158

lxxxvii https://www.forbes.com/2008/04/07/health-world-countries-forbeslife-cx_avd_0408health.html#3b2118763b11

lxxxviii https://www.ncbi.nlm.nih.gov/pubmed/28687259

lxxxix https://alivitycare.com/sauna-bathing-is-inversely-associated-with-dementia-and-alzheimers-disease-in-middle-aged-finnish-men/

xc https://www.ncbi.nlm.nih.gov/pubmed/30400288

xci https://www.ncbi.nlm.nih.gov/pubmed/15141356

xcii https://www.ncbi.nlm.nih.gov/pmc/articles/PMC4422005/

xciii http://www.jneurosci.org/content/25/11/2977

xciv https://medium.com/oxford-university/the-amazing-phenomenon-of-muscle-memory-fb1cc4c4726

xcv https://www.scientificamerican.com/article/mental-downtime/

xcvi https://www.ncbi.nlm.nih.gov/pmc/articles/PMC4492928/

xcvii https://en.wikipedia.org/wiki/Hermann_Ebbinghaus

xcviii https://www.ncbi.nlm.nih.gov/pmc/articles/PMC4492928/

xcix https://escholarship.org/uc/item/0kp5q19x

c https://www.ncbi.nlm.nih.gov/pubmed/30556597

ci https://www.ncbi.nlm.nih.gov/pubmed/23768180

cii https://www.ncbi.nlm.nih.gov/pubmed/26806041

ciii https://www.ncbi.nlm.nih.gov/pubmed/26147711

civ https://www.ncbi.nlm.nih.gov/pubmed/22725836

cv https://www.ncbi.nlm.nih.gov/pubmed/17987447

cvi https://www.ncbi.nlm.nih.gov/pubmed/28427563

cvii https://www.ncbi.nlm.nih.gov/pubmed/28852397

cviii https://www.ncbi.nlm.nih.gov/pubmed/2288601

cix https://www.ncbi.nlm.nih.gov/pubmed/12479842

cx https://www.ncbi.nlm.nih.gov/pubmed/29605221

cxi https://www.ncbi.nlm.nih.gov/pubmed/22336816

cxii https://www.ncbi.nlm.nih.gov/pubmed/28758188

cxiii https://www.ncbi.nlm.nih.gov/pubmed/28807434

cxiv https://www.ncbi.nlm.nih.gov/pubmed/19737808

cxv https://www.ncbi.nlm.nih.gov/pubmed/11687119

cxvi https://www.ncbi.nlm.nih.gov/pubmed/24354019

cxvii https://www.ncbi.nlm.nih.gov/pubmed/16437436

cxviii https://www.ncbi.nlm.nih.gov/pubmed/28421789

cxix https://www.ncbi.nlm.nih.gov/pubmed/30056419

cxx https://www.ncbi.nlm.nih.gov/pubmed/29703769

cxxi https://www.ncbi.nlm.nih.gov/pubmed/29310724

cxxii https://www.ncbi.nlm.nih.gov/pubmed/30513714

cxxiii https://www.ncbi.nlm.nih.gov/pubmed/30215171

cxxiv https://www.ncbi.nlm.nih.gov/pubmed/25463069

cxxv https://www.ncbi.nlm.nih.gov/pubmed/30081996

cxxvi https://www.ncbi.nlm.nih.gov/pubmed/28867798

cxxvii https://www.ncbi.nlm.nih.gov/pubmed/29268059

cxxviii https://www.ncbi.nlm.nih.gov/pubmed/28466678

cxxix https://www.ncbi.nlm.nih.gov/pubmed/27977429

cxxx https://www.ncbi.nlm.nih.gov/pubmed/30174138

cxxxi https://www.ncbi.nlm.nih.gov/pubmed/28418065

cxxxii https://www.ncbi.nlm.nih.gov/pubmed/30599760

cxxxiii https://www.ncbi.nlm.nih.gov/pubmed/30092587

cxxxiv https://www.ncbi.nlm.nih.gov/pubmed/29182711

cxxxv https://www.ncbi.nlm.nih.gov/pubmed/30551603

cxxxvi https://www.ncbi.nlm.nih.gov/pmc/articles/PMC2773815/

cxxxvii https://www.ncbi.nlm.nih.gov/pmc/articles/PMC4021146/

cxxxviii https://www.medicalnewstoday.com/articles/322648.php

cxxxix https://www.brainhq.com/

cxl https://www.mindgames.com/Memory+Games (Short term memory, You Won't Do Well level) cxli http://freebrainagegames.com/result.html

cxlii https://www.theatlantic.com/science/archive/2016/10/the-weak-evidence-behind-brain-training-games/502559/

cxliii http://visiontherapyblog.com/fun-online-games-to-boost-visual-skills/

cxliv https://journals.sagepub.com/doi/abs/10.1177/1529100616661983?forwardService=showFullText&tokenAccess=hK6Y5zBl1Rv.M&tokenDomain=rbtfl&journalCode=psia

cxlv https://www.pnas.org/content/113/27/7470

cxlvi https://www.ncbi.nlm.nih.gov/pmc/articles/PMC6153377/

cxlvii https://www.manchester.ac.uk/discover/news/human-brain-supercomputer-with-1million-processors-switched-on-for-first-time/

cxlviii https://archive.nytimes.com/www.nytimes.com/books/97/08/03/lifetimes/white-katharine.html?module=inline

cxlix https://www.newyorker.com/magazine/2005/02/14/andy

cl https://www.theatlantic.com/health/archive/2014/11/the-dutch-village-where-everyone-has-dementia/382195/

cli https://jamanetwork.com/journals/jamainternalmedicine/fullarticle/2587084#ioi160089r10

clii https://www.ncbi.nlm.nih.gov/pubmed/26863354

cliii https://www.alz.co.uk/alois-alzheimer

cliv https://www.ncbi.nlm.nih.gov/pmc/articles/PMC3096735/

clv https://www.ncbi.nlm.nih.gov/pmc/articles/PMC3096735/

clvi https://www.ncbi.nlm.nih.gov/pubmed/29653606

clvii https://www.ncbi.nlm.nih.gov/pubmed/30329009

clviii https://www.ncbi.nlm.nih.gov/pmc/articles/PMC2981103/

[clix] https://www.ncbi.nlm.nih.gov/pubmed/5084139

[clx] https://www.ncbi.nlm.nih.gov/pubmed/28851777

99

[clix] https://www.ncbi.nlm.nih.gov/pubmed/5084139

[clx] https://www.ncbi.nlm.nih.gov/pubmed/28851777

99